BASIC INDUSTRIAL HEARING CONSERVATION

BASIC INDUSTRIAL HEARING CONSERVATION

David F. Barr, Ph.D.
and Richard K. Miller

PUBLISHERS OF TECHNICAL AND SAFETY BOOKS
THE FAIRMONT PRESS, INC.
134 PEACHTREE STREET, SUITE 918 • ATLANTA, GEORGIA 30303 • (404) 876-1113

BASIC INDUSTRIAL HEARING CONSERVATION

Library of Congress Catalogue Card Number 78-74901
ISBN 0-915586-10-X

This book is dedicated to
David M. Lipscomb
Thomas A. Mullin
Cecil E. Kline
Pioneers in the field of hearing conservation.

Contents

1

NOISE: The Problem

Excessive noise that is physically and psychologically damaging to humans is largely a modern technological phenomenon. Having placed a "modern" time-frame on the problem does not negate the disturbance or annoyance factors in man's environment that surely existed from ancient times to the present. It is little wonder that the Roman poet, Horace, complained of the early morning clatter of chariot wheels on Roman streets. Damaging noise, however, is mainly an early nineteenth century problem. Prior to that time societies were in the main agricultural. New conditions of life were created with the industrial revolution: air and water pollution, waste products, worker exploitation and, of course, noise.

The energy sources necessary to maintain this "revolution" were coal, steam, oil and the toil of human beings. Coal, and certainly steam, are of less importance today, but the human factor remains. It is this human factor, and the need to conserve human hearing, that this book is all about. The authors are concerned not only with how to set up a hearing conservation program in industry, but also with presenting a rationale in human, social and economic terms to help explain why such programs are necessary.

We have come to believe—especially during times of recession and economic uncertainty—in the paradox of life in technologically advanced societies, that advancement in our material well-being must almost always be accomplished by some diminution in the overall quality of human life. Perhaps this was more true in the nineteenth and early twentieth centuries. Then considerations by industry to control noise pollution were in their infancy. We have fewer excuses now. To a large extent we possess the technology and the expertise to conserve hearing. All we lack is the desire to do so.

STANDARDS

Occupational noise-exposure regulations of the U.S. Department of Labor went into effect for the first time on May 17, 1969. It states simply that under Section 50-204.10 of the Walsh-Healey Public Contracts Act–Safety and Health Standards, any business wishing to sell goods to the Federal Government valued in excess of $10,000, or services valued at over $2,500, must take certain steps to protect the hearing of their employees.

The Occupational Safety and Health Act of 1970 (84 Stat. 1590)[1] extended this regulation to cover some 55 million workers in "all business engaged in interstate commerce." Enforcement of this act rests with the Department of Labor, and more specific penalties for violations were spelled out in this act. Also specified are the instrumentation and methods of evaluation of the data obtained.

WHAT MUST BE DONE

The regulation states (in part):*

> (a) Protection against the effects of noise exposure shall be provided when the sound levels exceed those shown in Table 1-1 of this section when measured on the A scale of a standard sound level meter at slow response.
>
> (b) (1) When employees are subjected to sound exceeding those listed in Table 1-1, feasible administrative or engineering controls shall be utilized. If such controls fail to reduce sound levels to within the levels of the table, personal protective equipment shall be provided and used to reduce sound levels within the levels of the table.

---

*Unless otherwise stated, noise regulations contained in this book are taken from Part 1910 of Title 29 of the regulations, as published on page 10518 of the *Federal Register*, Vol. 36, No. 105, May 29, 1971.

Table 1-1. Permissible Noise Exposures

Duration per day, hours	*Sound level dB(A) Slow Response*
8	90
6	92
4	95
3	97
2	100
1½	102
1	105
½	110
¼ or less	115

(2) If the variations in the noise level involve maxima at intervals of 1 second or less, it is to be considered continuous.

(3) In all cases where the sound levels exceed the values shown herein, a continuing, effective hearing conservation program shall be administered.

Exposure to impulsive or impact noise shall not exceed 140 dB peak sound-pressure level.

Chapter 4 begins our discussion of hearing measurement techniques that may be employed to comply with these regulations.

ECONOMIC CONSIDERATIONS

We continually hear of direct and indirect costs of industrial noise pollution to industry. At the same time, we hear of industrial claims of prohibitive costs of compliance to proposed standards of the Occupational Safety and Health Administration (OSHA).[3] Let us analyze some of these direct and indirect costs for you so that you might better see the reasoning behind hearing conservation programs.

The most obvious direct cost to industry is Workmen's Compensation claims for compensable noise-induced hearing loss. Joseph H. Hafkenschiel,[4] Economist for the Communications Workers of America, recently reported before the Senate Select Committee on Small Business, that the number of workman's compensation claims in California increased from 86 in 1955 to

620 in 1970, (a compound annual growth rate of 14%). The average award paid for noise induced loss in all states is probably around $2,000. (The average award in 1974 was $2,656 in Oregon and $2,504 in Wisconsin.) It has been estimated that at least 6 million workers suffer hearing loss due to excessive noise exposure. If we multiply these 6 million workers by the average claim of $2,000, we arrive at a potential workman's compensation liability of $12 billion. Let us compare this $12 billion figure with the estimated cost of a comprehensive hearing conservation program for industry which, of course, is another direct cost to industry of excessive noise levels. Estimates of audiometric testing programs, ear protection devices, technical audiological and medical supervision of the programs, and the paid time for hearing tests—audiological interpretation and testing and otological examinations—would cost at least $15.00 per employee per year. If we were to assume 10 million workers were overexposed to noise and included in our hearing conservation program we arrive at a figure of $150 million.

It is evident, therefore, that a reduction in excessive noise levels and the implementation of hearing conservation programs would not even come close in cost to the potential claims for noise induced hearing loss through workmen's compensation.

There are many indirect costs to industry as well which stem from excessive noise levels. These costs include those associated with excessive absenteeism, increased accidents and reduced worker efficiency and productivity.

Hafkenschiel[4] states that data from the iron and steel industry indicate that the increase in overall absenteeism among workers in noisy areas compared to non-noisy areas is 1.23 workers per hundred per day. If we use this rate and then apply it to the 10 million overexposed workers and assuming an average hourly pay rate of $4.50, the direct payroll cost of absenteeism due to noise may be in excess of $1 billion annually. This amount, of course, does not include fringe benefits paid to absent workers, overtime pay to compensate for loss of scheduled output per shift, or poor quality or defective products due to the absence of key personnel.

Noise is also a contributing factor in industrial accidents. In the previously mentioned study of the iron and steel industry, 35% of workers in noisy areas had 15 or more accidents in a five-year period compared with fewer than 5% in quieter areas.

Noise is a contributing factor in chronic and stress-related illnesses such as hypertension and alcoholism and contributes to increased production errors due to adverse effects on tasks requiring concentration.

Because we do not yet recognize the total costs to society of products produced in noise, their prices are artificially low. It therefore becomes evident that it is the worker who must bear the burden of industrial noise pollution. Hafkenschiel[4] states that "the theoretical optimal limit for occupational noise exposure will be that level which imposes costs of compliance in industry equal to the total cost to society of excessive occupational noise levels (and, thus, the total benefit to society of reducing them)."

The OSHA mandate to "preserve our human resources" thus becomes an economic as well as a moral imperative.

REFERENCES

1. Public Law 91-596. Occupational Safety and Health Act of 1970. 91st Congress, S.2193, Dec. 29, 1970. U.S. Government Printing Office, Washington, D.C., 1974.
2. Criteria for Recommended Standard . . . Occupational Exposure to Noise, National Institute for Occupational Safety and Health, Health Services and Mental Health Administration, Dept. of H.E.W., 1972.
3. Occupational Noise Exposure–Proposed Requirements and Procedures. OSHA Dept. of Labor, *Federal Register,* 39(27):37773–37778, 1974.
4. Hafkenschiel, J. H., Statement before the Subcommittee on Government Regulations, Select Committee on Small Business. U.S. Senate, Washington, D.C., July 24, 1975.

2

The Nature of Sound

Sound is a disturbance which propagates through a medium having the properties of inertia (mass) and elasticity. The medium by which audible sound is transmitted is air.

The propagation of sound may best be visualized by considering a vibrating object, as shown in Figure 2-1. As the object moves forward, it compresses the layer of air in contact with it. This compression travels outward as a sound wave. As the vibrating object moves in the reverse direction, the surrounding air is rarefied. This rarefaction travels outward in a manner similar to the compression. The result is a series of alternating compressions and rarefactions, in sympathy with the vibrations.

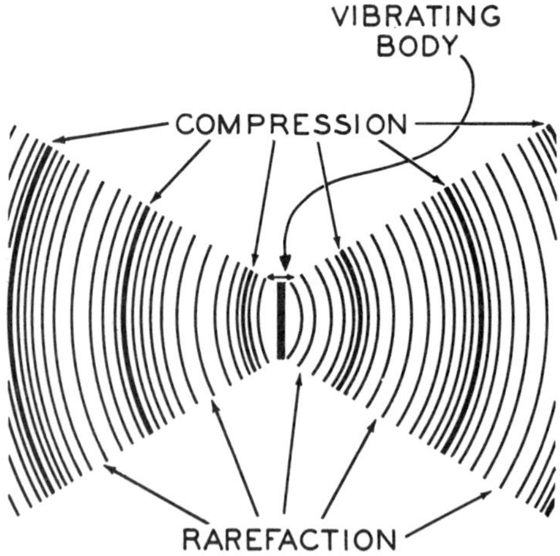

Fig. 2-1. Propagation of a sound wave due to a vibrating body.

The propagation of a sound wave may be depicted graphically by plotting the instantaneous displacements of the air molecules from their neutral position, as shown in Figure 2-2. The distance that a sound wave travels in one period or cycle is called the wavelength of the sound. The Greek letter lambda (λ) is generally used to designate the wavelength.

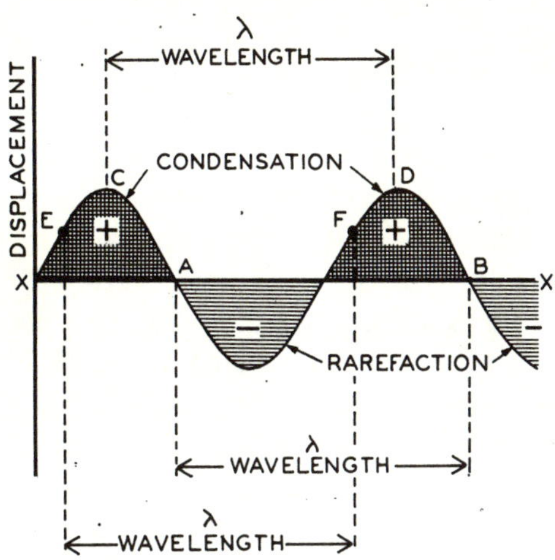

Fig. 2-2. Displacement-time graph of a sound wave.

The rate at which the molecular displacement of a sound wave occurs is the velocity of the wave. The velocity of sound in air at 70°F is 1128 feet per second. The velocity of sound as a function of temperature may be computed from:

$$c = 49\sqrt{R} \qquad \textit{Eq. (2-1)}$$

where: c = velocity of sound, ft/sec
R = absolute temperature, degrees Rankine
= 459.7° + °F
F = temperature, degrees Fahrenheit

The number of pressure cycles per unit of time defines the frequency of the sound wave. Frequency is perceived as the pitch of a sound, and is expressed either in cycles per second (cps) or Hertz (Hz).

The wavelength, velocity, and frequency of a sound wave are related by:

$$c = f\lambda \qquad \textit{Eq. (2-2)}$$

where: c = velocity of sound, ft/sec
f = frequency, Hz
λ = wavelength, ft

INTENSITY AND POWER

As with any energy source, the power of an acoustic source may be expressed in watts. In a free field, sound will propagate from a nondirectional source in a spherical manner. Since the area of a sphere increases proportionately with the increase in distance from the source, the intensity, or power per unit area, decreases because the power is being distributed over an expanding area. This is demonstrated in Figure 2-3. The intensity may be calculated from:

$$I = \frac{W}{S} \qquad \textit{Eq. (2-3)}$$

where: I = Intensity, watts/sq ft
W = Power, watts
S = Surface area, sq ft

The sound power level of a noise source is defined as:

$$L_W = 10 \log \frac{w}{10^{-12}} \qquad \textit{Eq. (2-4)}$$

where: w = acoustical power, watts
10^{-12} = standard reference power, watts

SOUND PRESSURE LEVEL

The sound pressure level in decibels (dB) may be defined as:

$$L_p = 20 \log \frac{p}{p_o} \qquad \textit{Eq. (2-5)}$$

where: L_p = Sound pressure level, dB
p = Sound pressure (rms), micropascals
p_o = Reference pressure = 20 micropascals

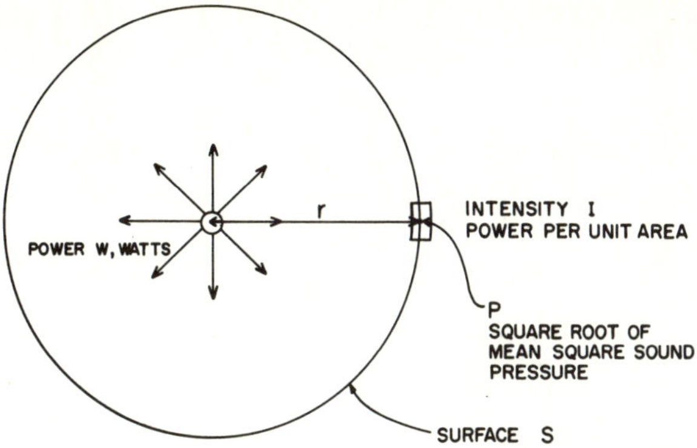

Fig. 2-3. Propagation of acoustic energy from a nondirectional source

The reference pressure, 20 micropascals, is the pressure equivalent of 10^{-12} watts/m^2, the threshold of human hearing.

Sound level meters are designed to respond to sound pressure, and are calibrated to read in decibels.

Table 2-1 presents the decibel equivalents for various sound pressures. In Figure 2-4, approximate decibel levels for various common noise sources are shown.

Table 2-1. Decibel Equivalents for Various Sound Pressures

Decibels	*Newtons/meter*^{2}	*PSI*
0	.00002	2.9×10^{-9}
20	.0002	2.9×10^{-8}
40	.002	2.9×10^{-7}
60	.02	2.9×10^{-6}
80	.2	2.9×10^{-5}
100	2	2.9×10^{-4}
120	20	2.9×10^{-3}

LOUDNESS

It is important to distinguish between sound pressure, a physical property, and loudness. Loudness is a physiological sensation. Since a sound of 100 decibels has an intensity of 10,000,000,000 times that of the threshold of audibility, it is indeed fortunate that our detection of sound is not linear with

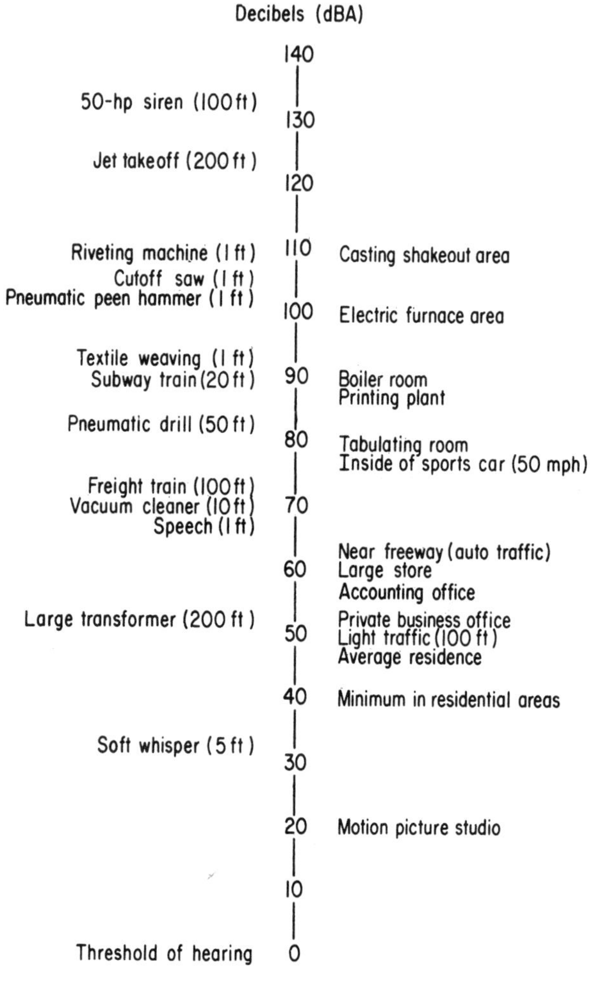

Fig. 2-4. Approximate decibel levels for various common noise sources

intensity. Table 2-2 relates changes in sound level to the average person's perception of loudness.

COMBINING DECIBEL LEVELS

Since decibels are a logarithmic function, they are not additive. For example, the combined sound level of two noise

Table 2-2. Subjective Response to Changes in Sound Level

Change in Sound Level	*Change in Loudness*
1 dB	Requires close attention to notice
3 dB	Barely perceptible
5 dB	Quite noticeable
10 dB	Dramatic; nearly twice or half as loud
20 dB	Striking, fourfold change

sources of 90 decibels each would not be 180 decibels, but rather 93 decibels. Table 2-3 may be used to combine decibels. To use the table, the difference between decibel levels is computed, and an adjustment factor is added to the higher level to determine the total sound level. To compute the resulting sound level when more than two sources are involved, the resulting sound from any two sources may be first computed. Then proceed computing the resulting sound level from additional pairs of levels until the final sound level is determined. This procedure is demonstrated in Figure 2-5 for the combination of six levels.

Table 2-3. Addition of Decibels

Difference between the two levels being added, dB	*Increment to be added to higher level, dB*
0 or 1	3
2 or 3	2
4 to 8	1
9 or more	0

OCTAVE BANDS

A sound level meter uses filters to determine noise levels for various frequency bands. The standard distribution is composed of 10 octaves. An octave band is a frequency range with the ratio of 2:1 between its high and low frequencies. The octave bands and associated center frequencies are listed in Table 2-4.

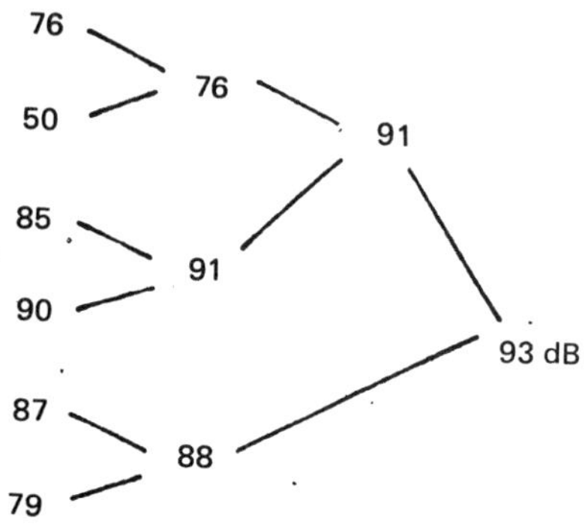

Fig. 2-5. Demonstration of procedure for finding the resulting sound level from combining the individual levels of 76 dB, 50 dB, 85 dB, 90 dB, 87 dB, and 79 dB.

Table 2-4. Standard Octave Bands

Center Frequency, Hz	*Octave Band, Hz*
31.5	22 – 44
63	44 – 88
125	88 – 177
250	177 – 355
500	355 – 710
1000	710 – 1420
2000	1420 – 2840
4000	2840 – 5680
8000	5680 – 11,360
16,000	11,360 – 22,720

– Hz refers to the frequency in cycles per second –

WEIGHTING NETWORK

While the human ear can hear sounds from about 20 Hz to 20,000 Hz, it is most sensitive to middle and high frequency noise. For example, the ear would perceive a 70 dB sound of 1000 Hz to be as loud as a 100 dB noise of 50 Hz.

The hearing response to pure tones of the human ear was first described by Fletcher and Munson[1] in 1933. Figure 2-6 presents the equal loudness contours which they developed.

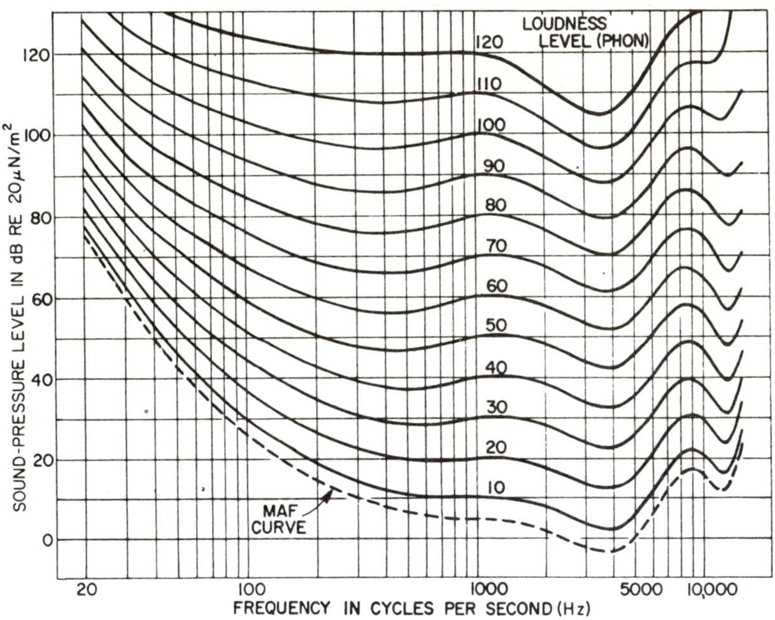

Fig. 2-6. Equal loudness curves

To provide the measurement of noise in accordance with levels actually heard by the ear, engineers have devised the "A-Weighting Scale." This weighting corrects direct noise levels to the levels heard by the ear. This corrected noise level is called a dBA, and is the unit specified in most legal regulations, including OSHA. To obtain dBA levels from octave band data, the adjustment factors of Table 2-5 must be applied. The A-weighting

Table 2-5. Conversion to "A" Scale Readings

	Octave Band Center Frequency, Hz								
	31.5	63	125	250	500	1000	2000	4000	8000
Adjustment Factor	−39	−26	−16	−9	−3	0	+1	+1	−1

curve approximately matches the 40 phon curve of Figure 2-6. B-Weighting and C-Weighting scales were also developed as shown in Figure 2-7. These scales weight the audible spectrum with more emphasis on the low frequencies than the A-Weighting Scale.

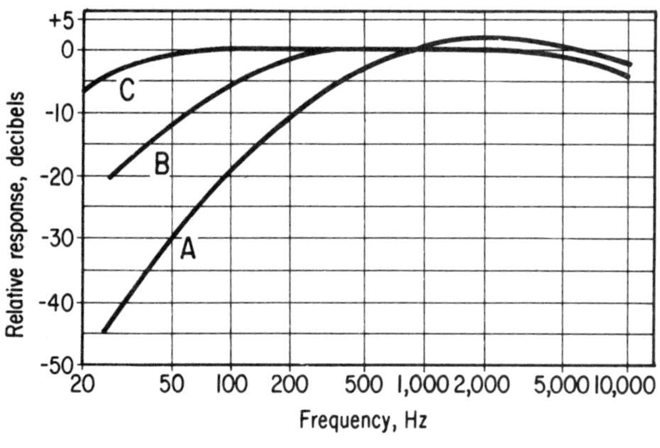

Fig. 2-7. Curves A, B and C are the international standards for acoustical weighting networks. The A weighting provides a frequency response that is similar to the human ear's.

REFERENCE

1. Fletcher, H. and Munson, W. A., "Loudness, its definition, measurement and calculation," *Journal of Acoustical Society of America,* 5 (2): 82-108 (October 1933).

3

The Hearing Mechanism

Hearing may be described as the humanizing sense, in that we develop those abilities that make us uniquely human—speech and language—through the auditory mechanism. The fact that the human hearing mechanism can be conveniently segmented and detailed for easier understanding, should not delude us into neglecting the great complexity involved in perceiving and processing the enormous amounts of acoustic stimuli necessary for us to become literate individuals.

The primary auditory functions may be divided into those involving acuity and those involving comprehension.

ACUITY

The hearing mechanism is the only 360° distance sense we possess. It never shuts off—being operative prior to birth—giving us a continual sense of connection with and protection from our our environment. Since our hearing never shuts off, it is heir to all the insults of our noisy environment. It is obvious that we can shut off our vision by simply closing our eyes, but we must invoke entirely different and more complex central nervous system (CNS) mechanisms to protect our hearing.

Continual noise of high intensity triggers protective reactions within the CNS, which attempt to attenuate the acoustic stimuli so that the hearing mechanism is thus free to concentrate on the more complex nuances of speech for learning and for communication to occur. A continual overloading of the system by noise inhibits the more complex functions of comprehension.

COMPREHENSION

Unlike acuity—which is primarily protective, directing our attention to the existence of sound—comprehension tells us what it is we are hearing. In order for understanding to occur, the auditory mechanism must be free from distracting influences. Should the auditory portions of the CNS continually attempt to produce ordered thought processes in the face of intense noise, it must do so only at the expense of the human being involved. See the non-end-organ effects of noise exposure in Chapter 5.

THE AUDITORY MECHANISM

For hearing to occur, acoustic stimuli must first find their way to the end-organ of hearing—the *cochlea.* This is accomplished first of all by sound entering the external ear canal, then through the mechanisms of the middle ear, on to the cochlea, and then to the brain stem and the auditory centers at the cortex.

THE EXTERNAL EAR

The external ear consists of the auricle or *pinna* and the external auditory canal. To the surprise of most lay persons and, unfortunately, many professionals also, the pinna serves more pragmatic functions other than as a structure merely to hang our glasses or earrings on. Gatehouse and Oesterreich[1] showed that the pinna transforms sound in such a way that permits humans to achieve relatively accurate monaural localization of the sound source, especially in conjunction with small movements of the head. Roser and Seipel[2] showed that the pinna is essential in the perception of median plane direction of the sound source. The pinna also attenuates low frequency noises, especially wind noise. It has a protective function, in that the cartilaginous tissue can absorb a great amount of force from a blow directed at the temporal lobe.

The external auditory canal or *meatus* (passage through bone) conducts sound to the middle ear. The canal contains fine hairs and cerumen producing (ear wax) cells. In combination these serve to keep foreign objects such as dirt and insects from reaching the *tympanic membrane* or ear drum.

THE MIDDLE EAR

The *tympanic membrane* or ear drum separates the external auditory canal from the middle ear. Sound strikes the ear drum and is transmitted across the tympanic cavity via the three middle-ear bones or *ossicles* to the oval window at the inner ear. The ossicles themselves are the smallest and hardest bones in the body. Should they be dislocated—as in a traumatic blast—a hearing loss as great as 60 dB may occur. These three bones are the *malleus* (hammer), the *incus* (anvil) and *stapes* (stirrup). Perforations of the tympanic membrane exert a variable amount of hearing loss, predicated on their size and location and whether or not there are associated changes in the middle ear. Losses range from a low of 5 dB to 20 dB in uncomplicated perforations.[3] The action and displacement of the tympanic membrane and the ossicular drain help to overcome the impedance—mismatch of sound transmission from the air medium of the external and middle ear areas to the fluid medium of the cochlea. The transformer action of the middle ear, therefore, recovers about 27 dB of the 30 dB lost when sound passes from air to liquid.

The muscles of the middle ear do not play a major amplifying role in sound transmission; however, they react reflexively in the face of intense sound. The *stapedius* muscle (innervated by the seventh nerve) and the *tensor tympani* muscle (innervated by the fifth nerve) contract in loud, prlonged noise exposure and may diminish the sound intensity by as much as 10 dB. The strength and quickness of this protective reaction is quite limited in the face of prolonged, intense exposure due to adaptation (fatigue) and/or if the rise time of a sudden loud noise is faster than the contraction time of the muscle. See Figure 3-1 for the basic anatomy of the external and middle ear areas.

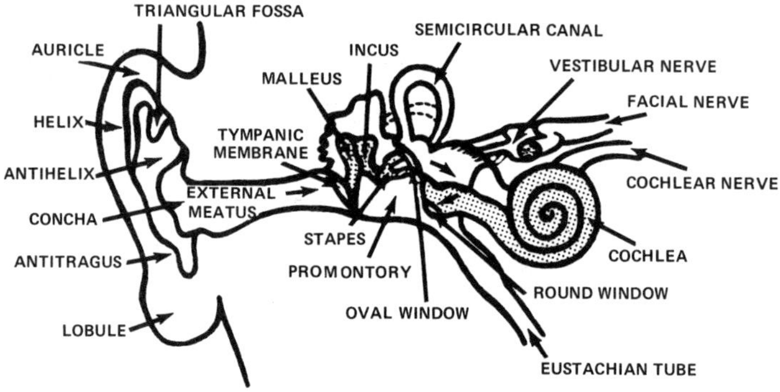

Fig. 3-1. Basic anatomy of the hearing mechanism[4]

THE INNER EAR

The inner ear is comprised of the end-organ of hearing—the cochlea, the organs of balance—the semicircular canals, and the acoustic and vestibular portions of the VIII cranial nerve. The cochlea itself has three divisions or *scalae.* The middle portion—*scala media*—contains the organ of Corti (see Figure 3-2). The fine hair cells, or *cilia,* bend selectively along the basilar membrane as acoustic simulation of the organ gives rise to electrical responses or firing of the hair cells. This electrical response is passed on to the temporal lobe of the brain by way of the auditory waystations of the brain stem and limbic system.

CENTRAL AUDITORY AREAS

The pathways of the central nervous system (CNS) are extremely complex, in that acoustic stimulation of cortical and subcortical areas can affect the functioning of the entire system. This fact will lead us to a more detailed discussion of the stress factors inherent in excessive noise stimulation in Chapter 5. Figure 3-3 features the main auditory junctions in the CNS.

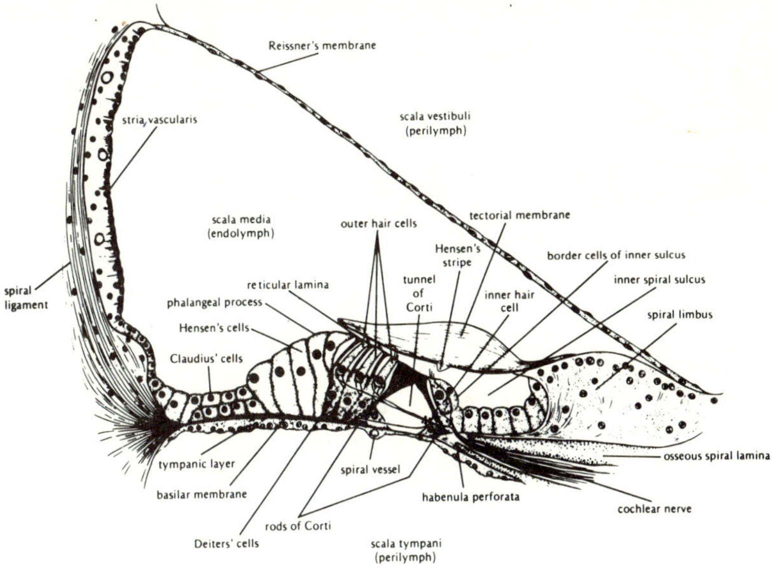

Fig. 3-2. A cross section of the cochlea showing the organ of Corti situated in the scala media on the basilar membrane.
(Drawing by Sarah Crenshaw McQueen, used by permission.)

The neural fibers from the auditory pathways ascend to the limbic system where information is evaluated as to its usefulness and/or danger to us. This information can be held in short-term memory storage until it is incorporated into long-term memory at the temporal cortex. Figure 3-4 shows the anatomical location of the limbic system. Figure 3-5 depicts the basic anatomy of the temporal lobe and the left cerebral hemisphere.

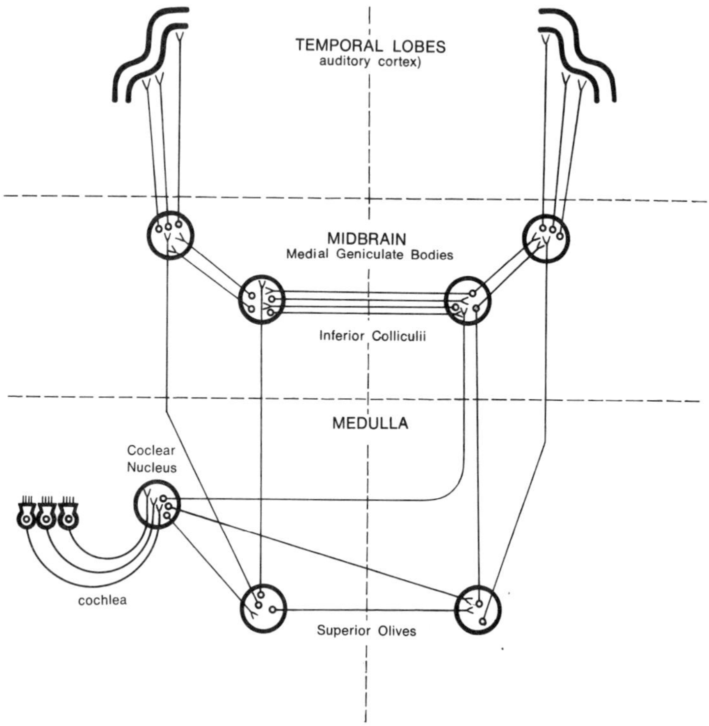

Fig. 3-3. Auditory pathway. Neural connections are shown for only one cochlea, but they are the same for both.[5]

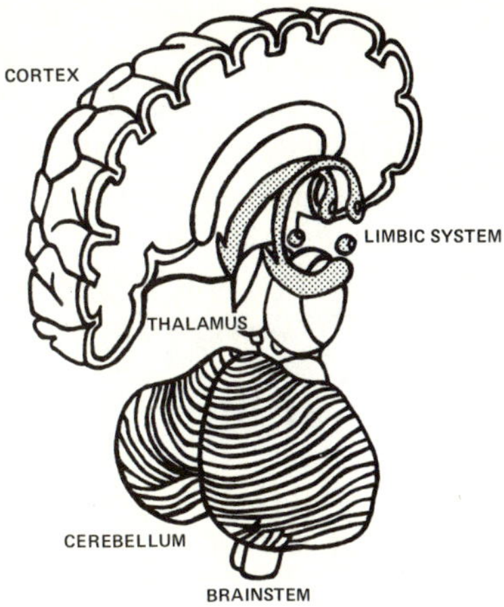

Fig. 3-4. Anatomical location of the limbic system[1]

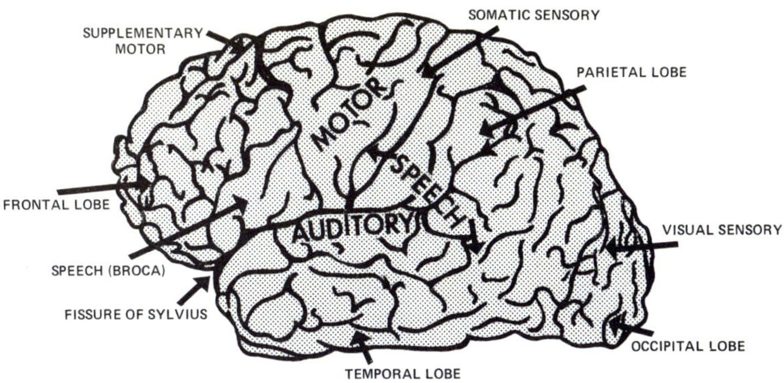

Fig. 3-5. Basic anatomy of the left cerebral hemisphere

REFERENCES

1. Gatehouse, R. W. and Oesterreich, R. E., "The Roles of the Pinna and the External Auditory Meatus in Monaural Sound Localization." *J. Aud. Res.*, 12 (1): 83-90, 1972.
2. Roser, D. and Seipel, K., "On the Formation of Directional Sensation in the Median Plane." *Arch. Klin. Exp. Ohr. Nas. Kehlk. Heilk.*, 205 (2): 256-261., 1973.
3. DeWeese and Saunders, *Textbook of Otolaryngology.* Mosby Company, 1964, 313-324.
4. Barr, D. F., *Auditory Perceptual Disorders.* Charles C. Thomas, Publishers, 1976.
5. Barr, D. F., *Auditory Perceptual Disorders: An Introduction.* Charles C. Thomas Publishers, 1972.
6. Johnstone, B. M. and Sellick, P.M., The Peripheral Auditory Apparatus. *Quart. Rev. Biophysics,* 5(1): 1-57, 1972.

4

The Measurement of Hearing

The human ear structure is so delicately tuned and balanced that sensitivity to acoustic stimuli covers a very broad range of 10 octaves in frequency and pressures near 0.0002 dynes/cm^2, at which point air particle movements are as minute as 10^{-10} cm. Over and above this extreme sensitivity range, the ear can support acoustic pressures as great as 140 dB, or one billion times greater than the faintest detectable sound. It is only because of this great elasticity of the ear that we are able to withstand innumerable severe insults to the auditory mechanism which is the every-day lot of millions of American industrial workers.[1]

It is the function of audiometric testing to discover those workers who can no longer sustain insults to their auditory mechanisms so protective measures may be taken.

THE AUDIOMETER

The measurement of hearing in the industrial setting is usually accomplished through the use of a discrete-frequency manual, pure-tone air conduction audiometer. The limited-range, pure-tone air conduction audiometer is the preferable type of manual audiometer for industrial testing. Regardless of how complex or how simple the audiometer is, it has the same purpose—to measure hearing acuity at certain required frequencies.

Typically, the audiometer will have the following:

1. *On-Off Switch*—This is the power switch which turns on the audiometer. Usually a pilot light tells you that the instrument is on. Should the pilot light fail to burn, probable causes are improper plug contact with the electrical outlet or the fuse could be burned out.

2. *Ear Selection Switch*—It is important to be able to switch the tone from one ear to another. Since the right ear is usually tested first, the color red or the word "right" matches the right earphone. When the right ear has been tested, the switch is turned to the left or to the blue color that matches the left earphone. The receivers or earphones should never be dropped. Should they be damaged in any way, they should be replaced and recalibrated. Since the earphones are calibrated to their audiometer, they should never be used with another audiometer.

3. *Interrupter Switch*—This switch is used to present the tone signal. It enables you to regulate the duration of the test signal and to determine whether or not the subject is responding to the signals you are presenting.

4. *Reverse Switch*—Many audiometers have a reverse switch which makes it possible to interrupt the presentation of a continuous tone, or when normally "off," the tone is produced by pressing the lever. For industrial testing, it is recommended that the reverse switch be kept in the "off" position. In this way, the tester is able to control the length of the tone presentation and to vary the time interval between presentations in order to make certain the subject is actually hearing the test tone.

5. *Attenuator Dial*—This dial contains intensity numbers that usually run from 0 (zero) to 100 or more decibels. Naturally, the lower the number of decibels, the softer the volume of the tone.

6. *Frequency Dial*–This control is employed to select the frequency (Hz) of the tone presented. The lower the frequency, the lower the pitch of the tone presentation.

Other controls, such as masking, bone conduction, microphone, or speech circuits may be disregarded for industrial testing in compliance with OSHA standards. Be sure that any such controls are always in the "off" position.

METHOD OF HEARING MEASUREMENT

The testing of hearing requires skill, precision and attention to detail, remembering always that you are working with a human being. There are, of course, legal and medical ramifications to everything done by an audiometric technician. This means that the accuracy of the audiometric test is very important. The following procedure is not the only one that is employed, but it is the most reliable and efficient method:

1. Turn on the audiometer and check it biologically before testing. This procedure involves the testing of a person with a known, stable hearing loss, or one with normal hearing. Should this biological check result in a 10 dB difference at any frequency tested, the audiometer should be checked electronically for calibration. A log book should be kept with a notation covering the date, time and results of the biological calibration. This procedure is to be followed before you begin testing for the day.
2. Take an in-depth case history on each worker. If you are testing a worker one year following his initial baseline audiogram, do not assume that the historical facts will be the same. Changes occur in lifestyle, environmental exposure and aural health from year to year. (See Figure 4-1 for an example of an in-depth case history form.)
3. Seat the worker in the sound-treated booth with his back to the tester. He should be instructed to respond to a series of tones by raising his hand and putting it down each time he hears the tone. Finger raising or head

NAME ____________________
Address ____________________
City __________ State __________ Zip __________
Telephone __________
Sex _____ Age _____ Married _____ Children _____
Loud noise exposure in past 14 hours: Yes ___ No ___
Previous employment noise exposure: (company) (city) (dates) __________

____

Military: Branch _______ Dates _______ Noise exposure _______
Hobbies: ____________________
Explosives exposure: Yes __ No __ Where _______ When _______
Rock music exposure: Yes __ No __ Where _______ When _______
Hearing problems in family: parents _______ brothers or sisters _______
General health: good ___ fair __ poor __
Diseases: Measles ___ Mumps ___ Typhoid ___ Scarlet Fever ___
Malaria ___ Pneumonia ___ Others __________
Medication taken: Streptomycin ___ Quinine ___ Others _______
Ear infections: Yes ___ No ___ Dates _____ Doctor _______
Dizziness: Yes ___ No ___ Ringing in ears: Yes ___ No ___ Dates _____
Above information is correct & complete _______________
SIGNATURE

Fig. 4-1. Case History Form

nodding are not acceptable responses. It does not matter which hand he uses, nor does it matter if he designates which ear he hears the tone in. The technician should know to which ear he or she is presenting the tone. Asking the worker to designate to which ear the tone has lateralized only takes time and can confuse the worker. Be sure the worker understands the instructions. Keep it simple.

4. Place the earphones on the worker, one ear at a time, with the headband across the top of the head. Should a female worker have on a wig or elaborate hairdo, crush the hair or wig down with the headband. Don't worry about messing up anyone's hair. The important consideration is proper placement of the earphones with the receiver or opening unobstructed and directly opposite the external canal of the ear. Large earrings should be removed prior to earphone placement. Do not test any worker with his hearing aid on. Have him remove it and turn it off. Note on his case history form the type of

hearing aid it is (behind-the-ear, all-in-the-ear, body-type, etc.), at which ear it is worn, for how long it has been worn, and with what success he has worn it.

5. Close the booth door and seat yourself behind the audiometer. Pick up your red and blue pen, turn the frequency dial to 1000 Hz at the right ear at 40 dB on the attenuator dial. Depress the interrupter switch for no more than one second. If the worker responds, lower the intensity by 10 dB and give the tone again until he no longer responds. Following one no response, turn the intensity up in 5 dB steps until he responds again. If he has responded twice at the same intensity, take this reading as threshold at that particular frequency and record it on the audiogram. Place the numerical reading in the appropriate square if you are using the block audiogram (see Figure 4-2), or use the appropriate symbol (red 0 for right or blue X for left) if you are using the graph-type audiogram (see Figure 4-3).

   Test the following frequencies in this sequence, employing the above technique: 1000, 2000, 3000, 4000, 6000 (8000 is recommended but optional) and 500 Hz. Turn to the left ear and repeat the same procedure. After testing the last frequency at the left ear (500 Hz), turn again to the right ear and retest the right ear at 1000 Hz. This response should be within ±5 dB of the first response for test/retest reliability. If the retest score is greater than ±5 dB, do the entire test procedure again. Should you still not have test/retest reliability upon testing the worker for the second time, do not attempt to test him again, but refer him to an audiologist for further testing. See "When Not to Test" section in this chapter.

6. Open the booth door, take the earphones off and thank the worker for his cooperation. Do not give any test information directly to the employee at this time unless you are an audiologist or otologist. Usually the worker is informed by management in letter form of the condi-

HEARING LEVEL BY NUMBER IN dB							
	500	1000	2000	3000	4000	6000	8000
R							
L							

ANSI 53.6—1969

Fig. 4-2. Block-Type Audiogram

Audiogram Key

AIR CONDUCTION

O Right Ear (red)

X Left ear (blue)

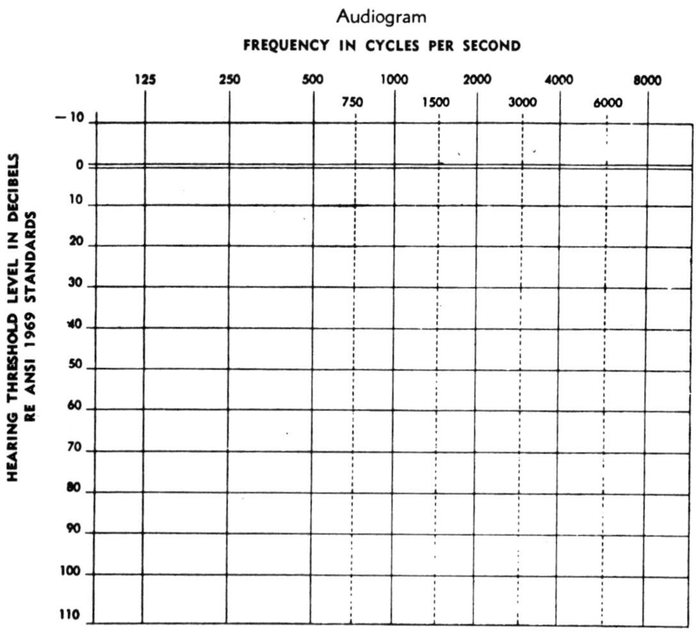

Fig. 4-3. Graph-Type Audiogram

tion of his hearing following professional review and recommendations by an audiologist or otologist. Be sure that your audiograms are professionally reviewed and that recommendations made by them are followed. Regardless of OSHA standards, it is of little benefit to institute an audiometric testing program and add audiograms to the workers' files with no professional review. Medical/legal considerations should warn the prudent employer of the stupidity and danger of following this ostrich-like procedure. Under present OSHA standards, audiograms must be kept for five years after termination of employment.

THE AUDIOMETRIC TEST ENVIRONMENT

Most of the ambient noise in the environment is low frequency centered. Since the cushions on the earphones provide less effective attenuation of these low frequencies, it is usually necessary to test hearing in an acoustically treated booth. Such a sound-treated booth only attenuates the ambient noise level; it does not eliminate it.

The American National Standards Institute (ANSI) sets maximum octave-band noise levels inside sound-treated booths. Table 4-1 shows the maximum background noise levels that can be present outside the room while a valid hearing test is being conducted inside.

Table 4-1. ANSI Maximum Octave-Band Noise Levels for Sound-Treated Booths (ANSI S3.1 1960 "Background Noise in Audiometer Rooms").

Octave Band Center Frequency (Hz)	*Permissible Background Noise Levels*	
	Level Outside (dB) Max.	*Test Room Level (dB) Max.*
500	86	40
1000	93	40
2000	105	47
4000	118	57
8000	130	67

WHEN NOT TO TEST

The following is a list of times the audiometric technician is not to test a worker, but should instead refer him on for professional management.

Do not test if:

1. The worker refuses to let you test him. Remember his First Amendment rights. He does not have to let you do anything to his person he does not wish you to do. Respect his rights, but state on the audiogram that the worker refused to take the hearing test and get the worker to sign to this effect if he will. The rule of thumb is, get what you can. Also advise the worker's superiors of his negative decision. Usually they or the union can change his mind.
2. If the worker has an obvious drainage from the ear, or should a perforation be noted upon otoscopic inspection, do not test the worker but refer him to an otologist at once.
3. If the worker complains of dizziness (sometimes accompanied by nausea, vomiting, fullness feelings at the ears, and buzzing or roaring head noises—tinnitus), refer him to an otologist at once. This procedure should also be followed if the worker complains of a fluctuant hearing loss—he hears better or worse at various times.
4. If the worker has been exposed to noise of 80 dBA or more within 14 hours prior to testing, do not test him. Workers so exposed prior to testing must wear ear protection with suitable attenuation levels to comply with the 80 dBA level.
5. If the worker is obviously "faking" a hearing loss, or if he repeatedly cannot follow instructions well enough to give a reliable audiogram, don't fool with him. Refer him on to the professional trained to test such hard-to-test cases—the audiologist. Make no "file 13" diagnoses of "psychogenic deafness" or the like. Just state that the test-retest reliability was poor and refer the worker on for audiological testing.

6. A sudden unilateral (involving one ear) hearing loss with or without poor speech discrimination ability, should receive immediate otological attention.

MANUAL vs AUTOMATIC AUDIOMETERS

It is evident that the audiometric technician has greater flexibility regarding testing procedures and more control over the test situation when using the manual audiometer. ***Control*** is the key word here. The automatic audiometer has been touted by many as a quick and efficient method of testing hearing, with the worker himself recording his hearing threshold by depressing the button as long as he hears the tone and releasing it when he does not. But is this method quicker and more efficient than manual audiometry? The experience of the authors and that of other researchers indicates that in many instances it is not.

In a 1971 study,[2] Gosztonyi, Vassallo, and Sataloff investigated the audiometric results of 100 subjects (50 shop and 50 office) employed in heavy industry. Four modes of testing were studied, but the most pertinent one to our discussion was the data relative to automatic audiometry in which some results were classified "unreliable" due to one or more of the following four categories:

1. A bilateral lack of response by the subject when the hearing level is at full intensity;
2. Audiometric tracings indicating severe hearing losses at all frequencies;
3. Wide or erratic audiometric tracings throughout;
4. Lack of superposition of the audiometric tracings (where the technician had repeated the test on the same card).

Although all 50 office employees' audiograms were judged reliable, only 27 of the 50 shop workers were evaluated as completely reliable.

Rintelmann[3] reports that the automatic audiometer presents certain special problems that are not encountered with manual audiometry, and, as a consequence of the difference in techniques used in the two procedures, hearing thresholds greater than 10 dB difference can be obtained from a large number of industrial workers. He further states that perhaps 30% of the employees might be unnecessarily referred due to lack of agreement from year-to-year testing with automatic vs. manual audiometers, and that poor test-retest reliability of successive audiograms could obscure actual hearing threshold changes that might be due to excessive noise exposure. Figure 4-2 shows a manual audiometer in operation.

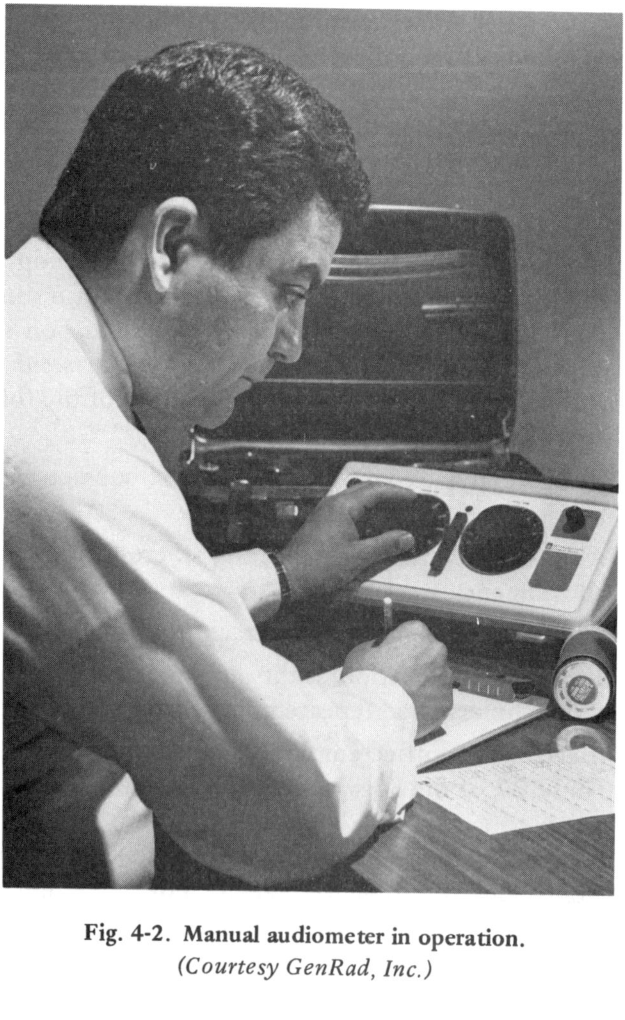

Fig. 4-2. Manual audiometer in operation.
(Courtesy GenRad, Inc.)

In that this chapter has indicated an obvious bias in favor of manual audiometry, it is only fair to mention that Robinson and Whittle,[4] in a comparison of manual and automatic audiometry, found the latter gave a mean threshold which was 3 dB more sensitive than the former at frequencies of 500 through 8000 Hz, while at 250 Hz there was no difference between the two techniques. Since these slight differences could arise from differences in threshold determination procedure, they concluded that the two types of audiometry gave essentially identical results.

Improvements in automatic audiometers, such as those found on Figure 4-3, are leading these authors to accept automatic audiometry for most industrial applications.

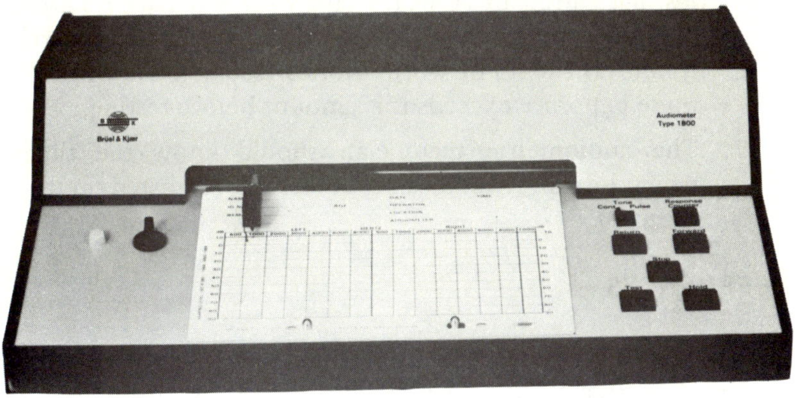

Fig. 4-3. Automatic recording audiometer
(Courtesy Bruel & Kjaer, Denmark)

GENERAL PROGRAM RECOMMENDATIONS

The following recommendations are designed to help management set up an effective, quality hearing-conservation program:

1. Either manual or automatic audiometers may be used.
2. The audiometric technician should be properly trained (see Appendix A for audiometric technician training).

3. All audiograms should be kept in a safe place where they are readily accessible. They should be kept for a period of five (5) years after termination of employment for each worker.
4. All audiograms should be reviewed by either an audiologist or an otologist, and their recommendations followed (see Chapter 5 for qualifications of hearing health professionals).
5. Audiograms are legal documents as well as medical records. No erasures should be made on them, and care must be exercised to insure accurate and reliable test results.
6. A 14-hour rest period is mandatory prior to audiometric testing. During this time the employee is to have no noise exposure greater than 80 dBA. Ear protection (generally muffs) should be worn prior to testing if the worker's noise exposure exceeds this amount before testing.
7. The audiometric technician should know the times when hearing should not be tested (as listed in this chapter).

REFERENCES

1. Harris, J. D., "Hearing Loss in Decompression." Report 591, U.S. Navy Submarine Medical Center, Submarine Base, Groton, Ct., 1969.
2. Gosztonyi, R. E., Jr., Vassallo, L. A., and Sataloff, J., "Audiometric Reliability in Industry." *Arch. Environmental Health*, 122: 113-118, 1971.
3. Rintelmann, W. F., "Manual and Audiometric Audiometry: A Comparison." *National Safety News*, 95-102, October 1973.
4. Robinson, D. W. and Whittle, L. S., "Manual vs. Automatic Audiometry Threshold Comparison." *J. Sound Vibration*, 26: 41-62, 1973.

5

Noise Related Hearing Disorders

It must be understood at the beginning of this discussion that when intense noise affects the auditory mechanism, the whole system is thus affected. There is no such thing as "pure noise-induced, sensorineural hearing loss" devoid of other profound CNS and systemic effects. Such thinking must be relegated either to the unsophisticated and/or the uninitiated.

Noise-related hearing disorders may be divided anatomically for physiological description of the impairment sustained.

Three factors influencing the onset of industrial deafness are:

1. The sound pressure level;
2. The total time of noise exposure; and
3. The susceptibility of the individual to noise.

CAUTION: NO EAR IS TOTALLY UNSUSCEPTIBLE TO PROLONGED EXPOSURE TO INTENSE NOISE.

THE MIDDLE EAR

Any hearing disorder involving the middle ear results in a conductive loss. A conductive loss is generally flat audiometrically or with the greatest amount of air conduction loss in the lower frequencies. See Figure 5-1.

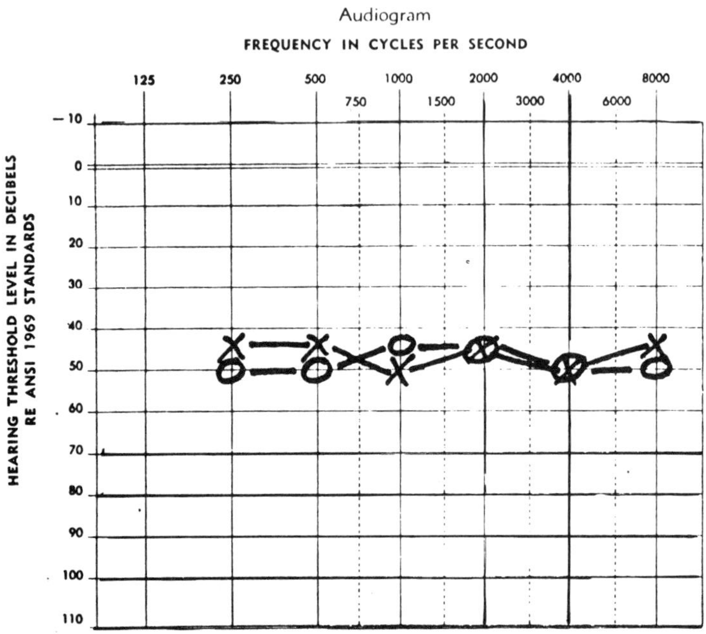

Fig. 5-1. Audiogram having a flat configuration with the hearing loss relatively constant at all test frequencies.

Some causes or etiologies of conductive hearing loss might be due to infection—called otitis media, perforations of the tympanic membrane, ossicular chain disarticulation, and eustachian tube dysfunction.

THE INNER EAR

Losses involving the cochlea of the inner ear are called sensorineural losses and are usually permanent in nature. Sometimes, as with a temporary threshold shift (TTS) after exposure to intense noise, the hearing threshold returns to its former level after a rest period of nonexposure. Such a return might only be cosmetic, in that many professionals in hearing feel that hair cell damage to some extent has occurred at the time of the threshold shift even though it returns to its former level audiometrically.

Noise induced sensorineural losses generally show a high frequency loss audiometrically. Such high frequency losses affect the ability to understand consonant sounds, and thus affect the ability of the worker to understand speech. This speech discrimination loss is best exhibited during the "cocktail party effect," when a lot of background noise is present, which interferes with speech perception. See Figure 5-2 for a typical high-frequency hearing loss.

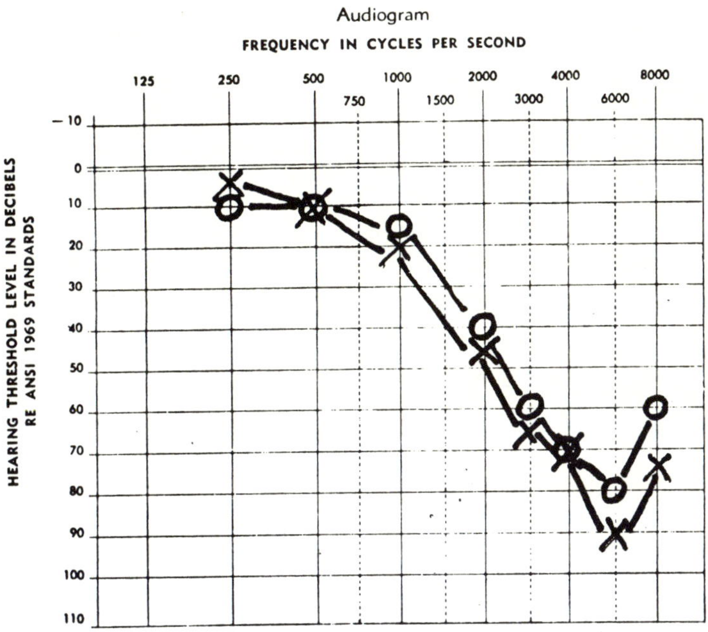

Fig. 5-2. Audiogram showing a high frequency loss configuration.

Frequently, following a great deal of initial exposure and/or exposure to a concussive noise, a high-frequency notch pattern can be seen, with the greatest amount of loss at 4000 Hz. This frequency—along with 3000 Hz—are most often involved in this noise-induced "notch" pattern. Figure 5-3 shows this configuration.

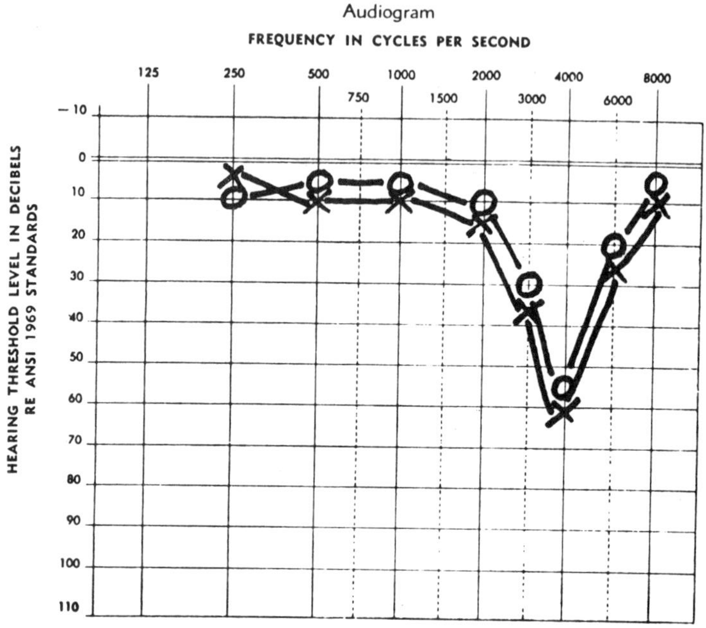

Fig. 5-3. Audiogram showing a typical high frequency "notch" pattern at 3,000 and 4,000 Hertz.

Almost all human inner ears examined, even those of teenagers, show some degree of degeneration of hair cells and nerve fibers in the basal or lower turn of the cochlea. This loss of sensory and neural elements appears to be a slow, life-long degenerative process which begins in infancy and culminates in the old-age hearing impairment commonly known as presbycusis. This process, common to all, can be greatly speeded up by exposure to intense noise.[1,2]

INNER EAR NOISE DAMAGE

Bohne[3] groups the wide spectrum of exposures that will damage the inner ear epithelium on the basis of their sound pressure level: very intense, intense and moderate. Actual SPL levels were not stated by the author, since levels defining each category vary from species to species, individual to individual, as well as frequency of exposure due to differences in the resonance characteristics of the external canal and the transfer characteristics of the middle ear.

Very intense—Damage due to the mechanical motion of the basilar membrane during exposure, which produces enough stress in the organ of Corti to cause rupture of its attachments.

Intense and Moderate—Exposures in the intense and moderate groups must be presented for several hours or days in order for injury to occur. One or more mechanisms other than mechanical are thought to be responsible for cellular damage produced by these lower intensities. Locus or maximal injury in the organ of Corti depends upon the frequency of the stimulus, with high-frequency sounds thought to damage primarily the basal turn with low-frequency sounds primarily damaging the apical coil. Based on the traveling wave theory of sound stimulation, damage may be far more widespread than formerly believed.

OTHER MECHANISMS OF DAMAGE

Metabolic Exhaustion—Damage to inner ear due to depletion of key enzymes and/or metabolites in the cells during prolonged exposure to noise.

Vascular Changes—Damage due to impaired circulation in the cochlear vessels during prolonged noise exposure. Such vascular changes may lead to a relative or absolute lack of oxygen and nutrients for inner ear cells.

Sonic Changes— There are two well-known fluids in the inner ear: Endolymph, with its high concentration of potassium (K+) ions and low sodium (Na+), is found in scala media. Perilymph, which is low in K+ and high in Na+, is found in scala tympani and scala vestibuli. Should noise exposure cause endolymph to gain access to perilymph through interruption of the reticular lamina, sudden changes in ionic content cause damage to the cells of the organ of Corti.

The audiometric technician is again cautioned against making clinical diagnoses of hearing losses from pure-tone air conduction data. Not even an audiologist nor an otologist would do so based on such limited test information. Figure 5-4 shows the degrees of hearing loss.

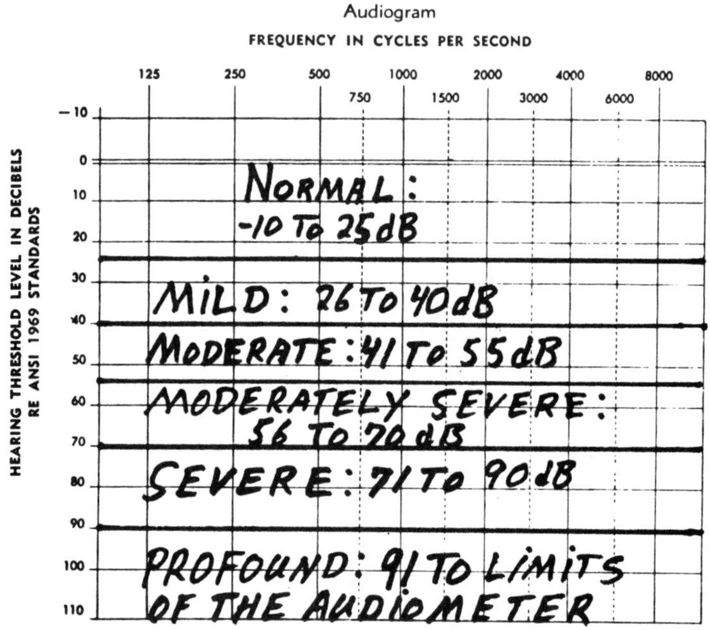

Fig. 5-4. Degree of hearing loss re ANSI 1969 standards.

CENTRAL AUDITORY AREAS OF CNS

Until recently little was known of stress-related changes in the CNS and the body due to noise exposure; as a consequence they were largely ignored or assumed not to exist. European researchers led the way with investigations by Jansen[4,5,6] who studied the effects of noise on the physiological state, and Grandjean[7,8] who investigated the biological background of noise related to the functioning of the reticular formation's nonspecific pathways to the brain. Investigations by American researchers were led by the definitive studies of Lipscomb,[1,9,10] Lipscomb and Roettger,[11] and by Cantrell.[12]

Early investigations on this most insidious and ubiquitous pollutant known to man, barred a true awareness of the nature and extent of noise effects on the CNS due to an arbitrary characterization of such "harmful" effects as being "only psychological." Overlooked in such "studies" is the obvious fact that temporary experimental noise levels do not truly simulate daily noise exposure environments. Not taken into account also was absenteeism, faulty workmanship and the physiological effects and family problems generated by offensive noise levels at work.[13] Chapter 1 discussed the economic aspects of these problems.

Westman[13] contrasts the government's attitude toward noise with its attitude toward drugs. Drugs under FDA regulations cannot be marketed without being proven safe for humans through prior laboratory testing on animals. In contrast the effects of noise exposure on experimental animals have for the most part been ignored. He further states that we now have enough evidence from animal studies to indicate that sound levels between 70 and 80 dB produce subtle long-range effects on humans.

ANIMAL RESEARCH

Following white noise exposure of 110 dB for 48 hours, Lipscomb[1,10] found exposed rats to have one or more forms of stress reactions: (1) shrinking of the thymus, which is a lymph gland just above the heart; (2) stress ulcers in the duodenum or other intestinal tract areas; and (3) swelling and discoloration of the adrenals, which are endocrine glands that produce carbohydrate-active steroids which act in an inhibitory manner in both the peripheral and central nervous systems in response to signals from the "master gland" at the brain, the pituitary. In this same vein, Henkin and Knigge[14] measured adrenal secretions of corticosterone in noise-exposed rats and found that their levels doubled following 30 minutes of exposure and trebled in 60 minutes.

Peterson et al.[15] studied the effects of noise on cardiovascular functioning in the Rhesus monkey. They concluded that noise may be one of the factors contributing to the long-term development of cardiovascular pathology in man. Of particular interest were sustained blood pressure elevations which may be induced by moderate but protracted noise stimulation.

Lipscomb and Roettger[11] found a reduction in the number of red blood cells in the auditory and balance sense end-organ regions in noise-exposed rats.

EFFECTS ON MAN

The myriad effects of noise on man are discussed only briefly in this basic text, concentrating on a few of the more dramatic recent research studies, in hopes of stimulating the interested reader to explore the more complete summaries of Lipscomb,[9] Schiff[16] and Cantrell.[12] See also Table 5-1 for a summary of noise-related disorders relative to anatomical areas of insult and/or their physiological functions in the auditory system.

Disturbing changes in brain-wave activity have been noted by Dieroff et al.[17] in his study of the relationship of EEG (electroencephalographic) measures to pure-tone hearing loss in 108 workers exposed to noise. Their results showed that 50% of the cases showed EEG changes with the onset of noise-induced hearing loss. There was a marked reduction in alpha activity (8 to 13 Hz; amplitude 30 to 50 mv), and a mixed type of alpha beta rhythm leading to a pure beta (14 ro 26 Hz; amplitude 5 to 10 mv) EEG. These EEG changes are present in the early cases of noise-induced hearing loss, and in the more advanced cases they are more frequent and more marked.

Cantrell[12] sums up the effects of prolonged exposure on man to intermittent noise as follows:

A. Healthy young men can live in an environment of intermittent noise in the form of a tonal pulse presented at 80 dB re 0.0002 dyne/cm^2 for 0.66 seconds every 22 seconds, 24 hours per day for 10 days without suffering major deleterious audiological, biochemical, or psychological effects; decrements in mental or motor performance; or interference with sleep habits.

B. When the noise is increased to 85-90 dB SPL, the noise becomes abrasive, and small but statistically significant decrements begin to occur in hearing and some interference with sleep habits occurs.

Table 5-1. Noise Related Disorders, Relative to Anatomical Areas and/or Physiological Functions in the Auditory System

Location	
Middle Ear	Conductive loss due to noise trauma (concussive sound). 1. Perforation of tympanic membrane. 2. Ossicular chain disarticulation.
Inner Ear	Sensorineural hearing loss at the cochlea. 1. Audiometrically usually seen at higher frequencies at 3000 through 8000 Hz. 2. Discrimination loss for speech—especially consonant sounds —due to damage to high frequency areas of the organ of Corti. 3. Vestibular problems and localization difficulties.
Central Auditory Areas of CNS	1. Stress due to Orientation Response (OR) and Adaptive Reaction (AR) in response to intense noise exposure, with rise in cholesterol and lower glucose levels. 2. Resulting decline in key neurotransmitters of CNS (norepinephrine and serotonin) and rise in monoamine oxidose (MAO) levels. 3. Reduction in brain alpha rhythm. 4. 5-HT concentration changes in amygdala of limbic system and temporal cortex (along with changes in other catecholamines) causing slow wave sleep interference (see 2 in this section).
Other Related Areas	1. Disruption of REM (rapid eye movements) time during sleep causing greater irritability, tiredness and difficulty in concentration. 2. Cardio-vascular changes (increased heart rate and vascular constriction). 3. Ulcers due to stress. 4. Motor coordination interference and difficulty in mental task performance calling for prolonged concentration.

C. At levels of 80 dB SPL, the blood cholesterol and plasma cortisol levels begin to rise significantly ($P < 0.01$) and continue to rise after exposure to 90 dB noise. Both levels begin to fall shortly after noise exposure is stopped. This presumed effect of noise has been shown in animals but has not been previously reported in man.

D. In assessing damage risk criteria for various noise exposures, the nonauditory effects of those exposures should be considered and measured.

E. Additional studies on the relationship of noise, stress, cholesterol levels and cardiovascular disease are indicated.

WHAT ARE WE REALLY MEASURING?

If we ask the above question within the context of present industrial pure-tone, air-conduction audiometry, the answer is obviously not much. When we consider the nonauditory effects of noise on man already discussed, it is equally obvious that we should be measuring a lot more than we do.

Even when we consider cochlear damage alone, the pure-tone audiogram does not reveal much about the condition of the sensory cells of the cochlea. Lipscomb[18] suggests that additional testing be done to assure that the scope and extent of inner ear damage may be more fully assessed for purposes of diagnosis, prognosis and rehabilitation.

Judd,[19] Nober[20] and Van Atta[21] point to the fact that the extent of hearing impairment depends on how you define impairment. The present 90 dBA standard for 8-hour expsoure is obviously too high by our current definition.

But what if we scrap our current definition based on pure-tone averages and 90 dBA exposure level?! Could we not shift from our present "damage-risk" orientation to a "noise-risk" orientation which focuses on the nonauditory effects of noise as well? Such a test battery would lead to a more complete and accurate assessment of the complete ramifications of noise exposure.

Moving toward a more comprehensive measurement of noise deafness prompted Noble and Atherley[22,23] to propose *The Hearing Measurement Scale.* They found that the degree of overall handicap suffered by someone with a noise induced hearing loss is mediated by their skill at lipreading. The acquisition of this skill is predicated upon the environmental factors extrinsic to the hearing loss itself and the visual acuity of the individual in question. They therefore propose a total speech perception ability assessment involving the testing of:

1. Pure-tone average (PTA) of the frequencies 1000–6000 Hz;
2. Speech discrimination score (DS);
3. Visual acuity tests; and
4. Lipreading ability.

The authors would propose a test battery incorporating ***The Hearing Measurement Scale***[22] along with EEG measures, blood cortisol and monoamine oxidase (MAO) levels. These measures would tell us the degree of stimulation of the pituitary-adrenal stress mechanism. Such a test battery could be termed ***A Noise Stress Index***. Such an "index" would give us far more information relative to the overall effects of noise exposure on man.

Yet to be explored fully and added to such an "index" are the effects on man of infrasonics (below 20 Hz) and ultrasonics (above 16,000–20,000 Hz).

In conclusion, we look to a new beginning of accurate measurements of the overall effects of noise and measures to control excessive noise levels in industry with these words by Lipscomb:[1]

> Audiometric and physiologic evidence to date do not indicate that noise in every form is dangerous to everyone. Conversely, no research evidence leads to the conclusion that exposure to excessive noise in any way facilitates human existence. It falls to students of the effects of intense sound upon man to distinguish between true factors that merit concern and mythical fears that result from inappropriate interpretation. Present evidence points to dangerous side-effects of noise stimulation and suggests it would behoove us to take prompt steps to abate excessive environmental noise.

REFERENCES

1. Lipscomb, D. M., "Living with Noise," *Hearing and Speech News*, 41(2):8-9 and 22-26, 1973.
2. Hawkins, J. E. and Johnson, L. G., "Patterns of Sensorineural Degeneration in Human Ears Exposed to Noise." In Henderson, D. et al. (Eds.), *Effects of Noise on Hearing*, New York, Raven Press, 1976.
3. Bohne, B. A., "Mechanisms of Noise Damage in the Inner Ear." In Henderson, D. et al. (Eds.), *Effects of Noise on Hearing*, New York, Raven Press, 1976.
4. Jansen, G., "Effects of Noise on Vegetative Nervous System of Man," *Ger. Med. Month*, 61:12-13, 1961.
5. Jansen, G., "Adverse Effects of Noise on Iron and Steel Workers," *Stahl. Eisen.*, 81:217-220, 1961.
6. Jansen, G., "Effects of Noise on Physiological State." In Ward and Fricke (Eds.), *Noise As a Public Health Hazard*, ASHA Report 4, Washington, D.C., 89-98, 1969.

7. Grandjean, E., "Physiologische und Psychologische Wirkungen des Laerma," Mensch und Umwelt. *Documenta Geigy*, 4, 13-42, 1960.
8. Grandjean, E., "The Biological Background of Noise Effects." In Ward and Fricke (Eds.), *Noise as a Public Health Hazard,* ASHA Report 4, 99-102, Washington, D.C., 1969.
9. Lipscomb, D. M., "Indicators of Environmental Noise,." In W. A. Thomas (Ed.), *Indicators of Environmental Quality,* Plenum Press, 1972.
10. Lipscomb, D. M., "Noise Exposure and Its Effects," *Scan. Audiol.,* 1(3):119-124, 1972.
11. Lipscomb, D. M. and Roettger, R. L., "Capillary Constriction in Cochlear and Vestibular Tissues During Intense Noise Stimulation," *Laryngoscope,* 83(2):259-263, 1973.
12. Cantrell, R. W., "Prolonged Exposure to Intermittent Noise: Audiometric, Biochemical, Motor, Psychological and Sleep Effects," *Laryngoscope,* Supp. No. 1, October, 1974.
13. Westerman, J. C., "The Human Cost of Noise Pollution," Statement before the Subcommittee on Government Regulation, Senate Select Committee on Small Business, Washington, D. C., July 23, 1975.
14. Henkin, R. I. and Knigge, K. M., "Effects of Sound on the Pituitary Adrenal Axis," *American Journal Physiol.*, 204:710-714, 1963.
15. Peterson, E. A.,;Augenstein, J. S.; Hosek, R. S.; Klose, K. J;, Manas, K.; Bloom, J.; Lovett, S.; and Greenberg, D. A., "Noise and Cardiovascular Function in Rhesus Monkeys," *J. Aud. Res.,* 15:234-251, 1975.
16. Schiff, M., "Non-Auditory Effects of Noise," *Trans. Amer. Acad. of Ophthal. and Otoloryngol.,* 77:384-398, 1973.
17. Dieroff, H. G.; Werner, R.; Stahl, T. and Reichel, G., "The Diagnostic Contribution of EEG in the Assessment of Noise Induced Hearing Losses," *Z. Laryngol. Rhinol. Otol.,* 52(12):908-914, 1973.
18. Lipscomb, D. M., "What is the Audiogram Really Telling Us? Part 1: Audiometrics vs Cochlear Damage," *Maico Audiological Library Series,* 13(5), 1975.
19. Judd, S. H., "Meeting OSHA Health Standards on Noise Exposure," *National Safety Congress: Industrial Subject Sessions,* 38-43, 1973.
20. Nober, E. H., "Noise Doesn't Just Harm Hearing," *Health & Safety,* 13-17, July/August 1974.
21. Van Atta, F. A., "Where is the Point of No Hearing Damage?" *Occupational Health and Safety,* 38-41, July/August 1976.
22. Noble, W. G. and Atherley, G. R. C., "The Hearing Measurement Scale: A Questionnaire for the Assessment of Auditory Disability," *J. Aud. Res.,* 10, 229-250, 1970.

23. Atherley, G. R. C., and Noble, W. G., "Clinical Picture of Occupational Hearing Loss Obtained with the Hearing Measurement Scale." In D. W. Robinson (Ed.), *Occupational Hearing Loss*, London, Academic Press, 1971.

For further information:

24. Calogero, B. and Vetrano, G., "Variations of the Biogenic Amines Content in Some Different Areas of the Brain of Rats Subjected to Physiological Auditory Stimulation and Acoustic Trauma," *Rev. Laryngol. Otol. Rhinol.*, 94(9-10), 429-443, 1973.
25. Lipscomb, D. M. (Ed.), *Noise and Audiology*, Baltimore, University Park Press, 1978.
26. Noble, W. G., "Critical Factors in the Assessment of Deafness Due to Noise," *Maico Audiological Library Series*, 11(8), 1972.
27. Salvi, R. J., "Central Components of the Temporary Threshold Shift." In Henderson, D. et al. (Eds.), *Effects of Noise on Hearing*, 247-260, New York, Raven Press, 1976.

6

In-Plant vs Contract Hearing Conservation Programs

Through the Occupational Safety and Health Act of 1970, the Department of Labor has established rigid guidelines for industrial noise control and hearing conservation programs. The new proposed recommendations[1,2] and the recommendations of the OSHA Standards Advisory Committee on Noise,[3] forebode of tougher standards in the future. Obviously management must assume the responsibility of showing that every effort is being made, through engineering, administration and hearing conservation programs, to prevent damage to the hearing of their employees. One method of providing an effective hearing protection program is through contract hearing conservation services.

The following is a list of advantages of such contract services:[4]

1. *Required Medical Surveillance.* The possibility of the existence of ear pathologies presupposes the need for medical surveillance and referral. For many plants, otological and audiological surveillance is not economically feasible and can be more cheaply provided through contract services. Such medical and audiological surveillance helps to prevent increased compensation claims at a later date by early and proper management of hearing problems.

2. ***Computerized Record Keeping and Analysis.*** The required audiometric testing of even a few hundred employees will generate thousands of audiograms in a short span of time. Professional processing of massive amounts of data is almost economically impossible without computerization. With computerized services less storage problems and increased retrieval ability is evident. Analysis of degree of loss and subsequent audiogram deviations from baseline readings are available in rapid fashion. The research potential of computerized data cannot be overemphasized. The research methodology and types of data collected in the occupational noise and hearing survey by Lempert and Henderson[5] points to the research potential of the four primary types of data collected during the course of an individual noise and hearing study whereby noise measurements, personal background information, medical and otologic data, and audiometric data are collected and analyzed.

3. ***Uniformity in Multiple Plant Operations.*** When the same data is collected on the same type of audiogram form, interplant transfer of employees presents no problem since records are the same.

4. ***Elimination of Problems of Turnover of Testing Personnel and Equipment Maintenance and Calibration.*** Contract hearing conservation services eliminate the problem of turnover of qualified personnel, the need to buy expensive audiometric equipment, and the expense of maintaining and calibrating that equipment.

5. ***Continuity of Analysis.*** Annual re-evaluations, with deviations computed from the original baseline audiogram provide a continuous check on the effectiveness of the hearing conservation program.

6. ***Unbiased Third-Party Administration.*** There is reason to believe that an unbiased third party giving evidence in compensation claims carries increased weight in court.

7. ***Minimal Lost Production Time.*** Many times the major cost to management in implementing a hearing conservation program is lost production time. In a contract mobile situation,

most companies can complete the testing and intake program in a minimum of seven minutes per employee using a manual audiometer.

8. *Engineering Assistance.* Engineering assistance for noise control is available through contract services that may not otherwise be available to many small- to medium-size plants.

9. *OSHA Compliance.* When a company contracts to provide hearing conservation services, that is often their only business. They devote their entire time to keeping abreast of new trends, laws and regulations.

10. *Expertise Transfer.* Much wasted effort in setting up hearing conservation services can be averted through the transfer of information from contract services to industry. Information on effective conservation programs, methods of procedure, policies and reasons for those policies can mean dollars saved.

11. *Economic Advantages.* When all the above services are combined into one package, in most instances contract hearing conservation services can be obtained at between 25% to 50% less than it would cost to provide these services in-plant. Of course, if a single plant employs more than one thousand employees, it is probably more economically advantageous to institute an in-plant program and then utilize the contract services' computer and record-keeping facilities.

It is not the intent to make expansive claims as to the efficacy of contract hearing conservation services for all of industry. But, given the limitations listed above, a contract hearing conservation service is the best solution for many small- to medium-sized plants.

IN-PLANT SERVICES

Plants who employ over one thousand employees working in excessive noise should set up their own in-plant services. This is so for the following reasons:

1. Given an average annual cost of $15 per employee for audiometric testing, and another $5 for hearing protec-

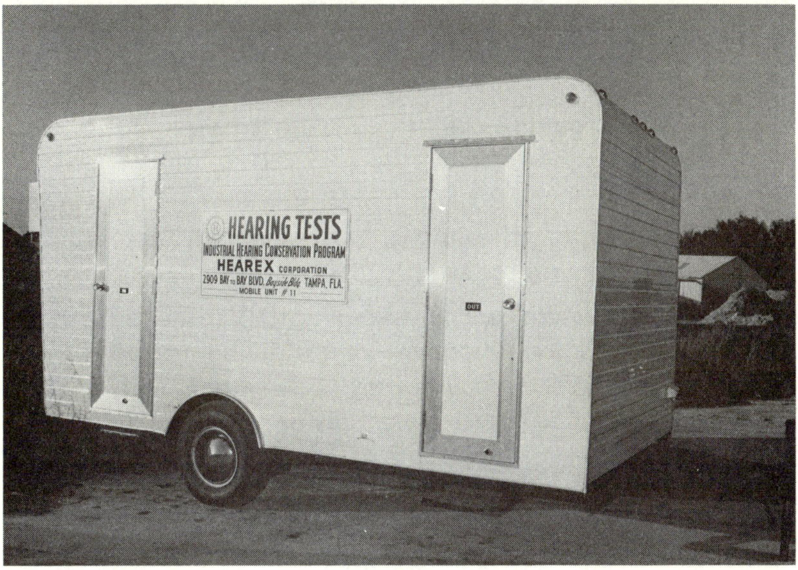

Fig. 6-1. Mobile facility for audiometric testing. Testing is performed within an audiometric booth located inside the trailer. Contract service companies utilize units such as this to perform on-site testing at industrial client facilities. *(Courtesy of Hearex Corporation, Tampa, Florida)*

tion devices, a full-time audiometric technician can be hired, and audiometric testing equipment purchased for less than the annual cost of providing hearing conservation services for 1000 or more employees.

2. With in-plant facilities for a great number of employees, a year round testing program can be instituted that is impossible for contract services to provide. With such a program, pre-employment and special retests (those requiring 3- or 6-month rechecks) can be handled all year long.

3. Closer supervision of the wearing of hearing protection devices, as well as continual emphasis on the need of such protection can be more easily accomplished for large numbers of employees with in-plant services. Con-

tinual and effective monitoring of hearing conservation programs involving large numbers of employees is essential.

SELECTING A PROFESSIONAL CONSULTANT

The initial choice is quite simple; you have but two groups trained to monitor an industrial hearing conservation program, otoloryngologists and/or audiologists.

Otoloryngologists are physicians (MDs) specializing in the surgery and medical treatment of ear pathologies. Few have direct training in industrial hearing conservation, and, as a consequence, should be screened carefully as to credentials.

Audiologists are scientists of hearing with broad training in the diagnosis and rehabilitation of hearing disorders. Audiologists have an M.A. or Ph.D. (a master's plus a clinical fellowship year is minimal) and are certified in audiology by the American Speech and Hearing Association. As with the otologist, caution must be exercised in assuming extensive training in industrial hearing conservation among audiologists. Most of them work in community speech and hearing centers, hospitals, or university settings and possess limited industrial experience.

HOW BEST TO CHOOSE

Either professional group can review audiometric results and make suitable recommendations. Ideally, one should possess certification as a program instructor by the Council for Accreditation in Occupational Hearing Conservation. This Council was organized to establish standards to evaluate and maintain the quality of occupational hearing conservation in American industry. A list of certified instructors may be obtained from the Council. For Council information contact:

Mildred A. Sittner, R.N.
1619 Chestnut Ave.
Haddon Heights, NJ 08035

DISADVANTAGES OF OUTSIDE CONSULTANTS

1. Many consultants operate without sufficient background in industry. Community speech and hearing clinics offering "free" consulting services in order to secure either testing and/or review of audiogram contracts should be considered with caution.
2. Many professional consultants are too busy with their practices, teaching schedules, research, etc. to give adequate time to industry. Be sure your consultant has enough time to serve your needs adequately. As Miller[6] has said, "Hourly fees are generally of only secondary importance; only the total fee and final results should be considered."
3. The consultant may lack familiarity with your plant operations. The time factor enters in here again. The consultant should become familiar with your plant and its product(s), as well as with your particular noise problems and hearing conservation needs.

ADVANTAGES OF PROFESSIONAL CONSULTANTS

1. The fruits of your hearing conservation program, e.g. audiometric results, will result in action being taken to insure the aural health of your employees. Hearing conservation programs which do not provide for professional review of their audiograms, and which do not provide for some system of medical and/or audiological follow-up for problem employees, are in essence providing no program at all.[7]
2. The consultant brings a degree of expertise not present among your staff. The consultant's suggestions should be weighed relative to your plant's needs, resources, and basic philosophy.
3. The experience of the consultant could be invaluable as an expert witness in contesting OSHA citations and work compensation cases involving hearing loss.

HOW TO DETERMINE THE NEED FOR A HEARING CONSERVATION PROGRAM

1. Review federal and state noise regulations.
2. Conduct sound level meter and dosemeter surveys in dBA (see 7).
3. If noise levels are all below 85 dBA, you have compliance and need go no further. Should certain areas have noise levels in excess of 85 dBA, proceed to 4.
4. Do you have personnel exposed to these noise levels? If no, document this fact. If yes, proceed to 5.
5. The extent of exposure to personnel must be determined. Does this exposure exceed the guidelines? If no, document this. If yes, proceed to 6.
6. Conduct an octave-band analysis of the sound source.
7. Are engineering controls feasible? If yes, implement. If no, document.
8. Are administrative controls feasible? If yes, implement. If no, document.
9. Develop and initiate a hearing conservation program.
10. Provide required hearing tests, and provide for their review and interpretation and storage.
11. Issue hearing protection devices in conjunction with an ongoing educational program (see Chapter 7).
12. Remember that an effective, ongoing hearing conservation program must provide for the following:
    a) Qualified personnel
    b) Appropriate record keeping
    c) Adequate test facilities
    d) Calibration and maintenance of all test equipment
    e) Baseline audiograms
    f) Annual retests, or as directed by professional consultants
    g) No exposure to noise levels greater than 80 dBA for 14 hours prior to testing
    h) Mandatory use of hearing protection devices
    i) Annual refresher courses for audiometric technicians

j) Review and continual update of hearing conservation testing program and changes in federal and/or state regulations

REFERENCES

1. *Guidelines to the Department of Labor's Occupational Noise Standards,* U.S. Department of Labor, Bulletin 334, Revised 1971.
2. "The Emerging New OSHA Noise Standards," *Occupational Hazards,* 38-42, July 1973.
3. *Recommendations of the OSHA Standards Advisory Committee on Noise,* U.S. Department of Labor, September 24-25, 1973.
4. Barr, D. F. and Kline, C. E., "The Advantages of Contract Hearing Conservation Services." Paper presented at the National Noise and Vibration Control Conference, Chicago, Illinois, June 1974, and published in *NOISEXPO Proceedings,* 1974.
5. Lempert, B. L. and Henderson, T. L., Occupational Noise and Hearing 1968-1972, *NIOSH,* Dept. of H.E.W., Cincinnati, Ohio, 1973.
6. Miller, R. K., *Handbook of Industrial Noise Management,* 171-180, Atlanta, The Fairmont Press, 1976.
7. Barr, D. F., "Hearing Conservation–The Moral Dilemma," *Sound & Vibration,* January 1975.

7

Hearing Protective Devices

Sound levels reaching the inner ear may be effectively attenuated by the use of hearing protective devices. Five categories of hearing protection are commonly used in industrial applications. The characteristics of these types are as follows:[1]

Insert (aural) earplugs are positioned within the external ear canal. They are available in various sizes in premolded form, as custom-fit units or as universal fit, disposable type items, consisting of materials such as wax-impregnated cotton, clay, glass wool, moldable plastic or sponge.

Semi-insert (semi-aural) earplugs are positioned against the opening of the external ear canal and are commonly suspended on a lightweight headband, but may also be self-retaining.

Earmuffs consist of two circumaural earcups on a retention system, with each earcup completely enclosing an external ear. The retention system holds the earcups against the sides of the head and is usually an adjustable headband worn over or behind the head, or under the chin. Earmuffs are also mounted on safety "hard hats," welding masks, helmets and similar items of personal equipment.

Supra-aural units which rest directly on the pinna and are usually designed for communication purposes, may also provide hearing protection.

Helmets cover a substantial portion of the head and may provide hearing protection; however, few helmets are designed with hearing protection as their primary function.

The attenuation characteristics of the various types of hearing protection are presented in Figure 7-1.

EXPECTED RANGE OF HEARING PROTECTION (ON AVERAGE) OF GOOD PROTECTIVE DEVICES					
HEARING PROTECTION	FREQUENCY RANGE IN HERTZ				
	1-20	20-100	100-800	800-8000	78000
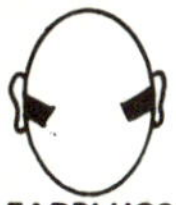 EARPLUGS	5-10	5-20	20-35		30-40
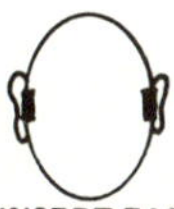 SEMI-INSERT EARPLUGS	5-10	5-20	15-20	25-40	30-40
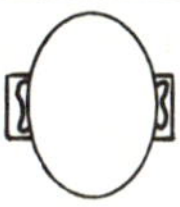 EARMUFFS	0-2	2-15	15-35	30-45	35-45
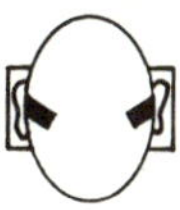 EARPLUGS AND EARMUFFS	10-15	15-25	25-45	30-60	40-60
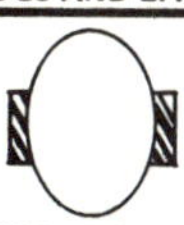 COMMUNICATION HEADSETS	0-2	2-10	10-30	25-40	30-40
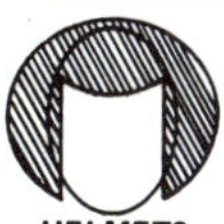 HELMETS	0-2	2-2	7-20	20-55	30-55
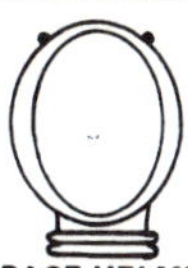 SPACE HELMET (TOTAL HEAD ENCLOSURE)	3-8	5-10	10-25	30-60	30-60

Fig. 7-1. Approximate maximum and minimum attenuation values, in decibels, for various types of hearing protection devices.[1]

The question is often asked: "Which devices provide the greatest attenuation, muffs or plugs?" Figure 7-2, from a recent NIOSH study[2] charts the mean adjusted attenuation for 48 earplugs and 102 ear muffs as a function of the (dBC-dBA) value. The results show that ear muffs provide slightly greater attenuation.

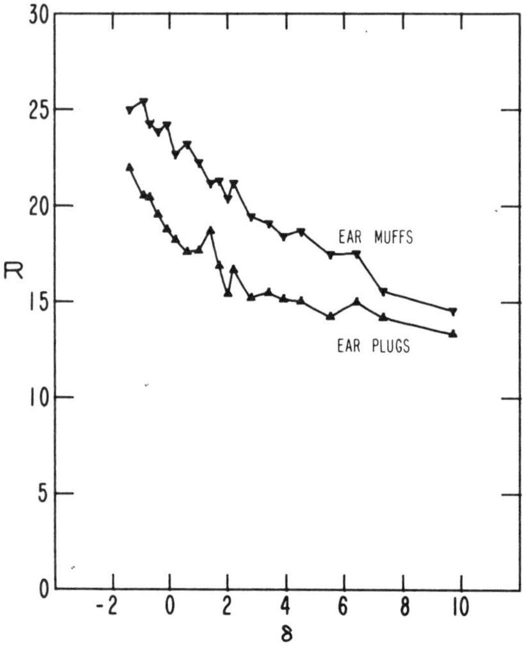

Fig. 7-2. Mean adjusted dBA-reduction factor (R) for 48 earplugs and 102 earmuffs as a function of δ (i.e. $L_C - L_A)^2$.

In general, most commercially available devices will provide effective attenuation for sound levels up to 105 dBA; many devices will provide an even greater attenuation.

A recent publication by NIOSH, "List of Personal Hearing Protectors and Attenuation Data," lists attenuation data for 175 ear protectors by 40 manufacturers. It is designated HEW Publication No. (NIOSH) 76-120, and is available from:

NIOSH
Office of Technical Publications
Post Office Building, Room 530
Fifth and Walnut Streets
Cincinnati, Ohio 45202
(513) 684-2723

LIMITATIONS OF PROTECTION

As shown in Figure 7-3, sound may reach the inner ear of persons wearing hearing protectors by four paths:

1. By passing through air leaks in the protector
2. By transmission through the protector
3. By vibration of the protector
4. By passing through bone and tissue around the protector.

Practical limitations for earplugs and ear muffs are shown in Figure 7-4.

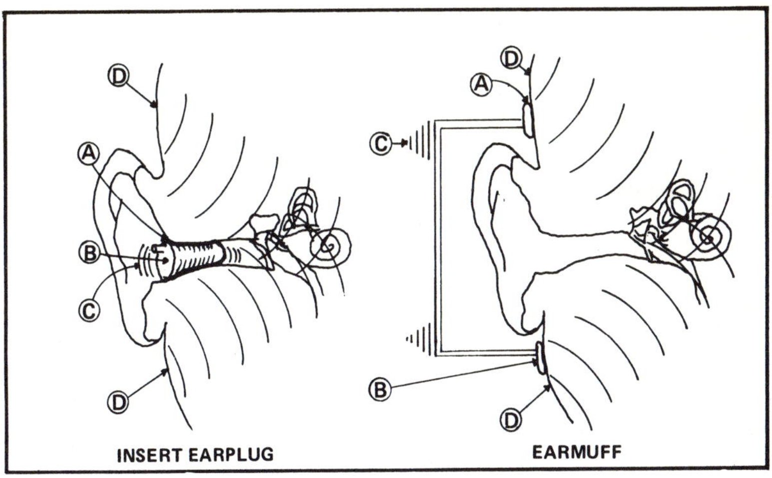

Fig. 7-3. Pathways of acoustic energy to inner ear while wearing protection. A–Air leak, B–Transmission through the material, C–Motion of the device, D–Tissue and bone conduction of head.[1]

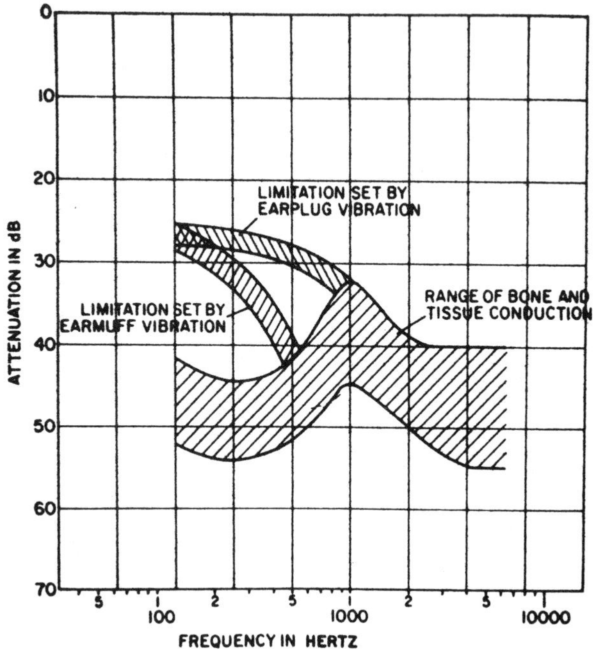

Fig. 7-4. Practical protection limits for plugs and muffs.[3]

TESTING OF DEVICES

Most hearing protection devices have been tested according to the American National Standards Institute (ANSI) standard Z24.22–1957 "Method for the Measurement of the Real-Ear Attenuation of Ear Protectors at Threshold."

Recently a new standard has been published which is a revision of the ANSI 1957 standard. The new standard is ASA STD1–1975 (ANSI 3.19–1974), "Method for the Measurement of Real-Ear Protection of Hearing Protectors and Physical Attenuation of Earmuffs." The main changes which are incorporated in the ASA 1975 standard are the substitution of third-octave bands of noise instead of discrete tones as the test stimuli, the replacement of an anechoic test room by a reverberant test room, and the inclusion of an objective method for measuring physical attenuation of earmuffs.

DETERMINATION OF NOISE REDUCTION

Three methods may be employed to calculate the noise reduction which is achieved by hearing protection devices based on manufacturers' test data. The methods result in an "adjusted dBA-reduction factor," denoted by "R." After R has been calculated, it can be subtracted from the measured workplace noise level (dBA) to obtain the effective noise exposure level for the worker. For example, if the measured workplace noise level is 112 dBA and the R factor has been calculated as 27 decibels, then the worker's effective noise level is 85 dBA.

In all three methods "Q" values are based on manufacturers' data of the mean attenuation and standard deviation of a particular hearing protector. The "Q" values are calculated as follows:

Q_1 = attenuation at 125 Hz, plus 16.2 dB, minus 2 X (standard deviation)

Q_2 = attenuation at 250 Hz, plus 8.7 dB, minus 2 X (standard deviation)

Q_3 = attenuation at 500 Hz, plus 3.3 dB, minus 2 X (standard deviation)

Q_4 = attenuation at 1000 Hz, minus 2 X (standard deviation)

Q_5 = attenuation at 2000 Hz, minus 1.2 dB, minus 2 X (standard deviation)

Q_6 = average of attenuations at 3000 and 4000 Hz, minus 1.0 dB, minus standard deviation at 3000 Hz, minus standard deviation at 4000 Hz

Q_7 = average of attenuations at 6000 and 8000 Hz, plus 1.1 dB, minus standard deviation at 6000 Hz, minus standard deviation at 8000 Hz

The numbers +16.2, +8.7, +3.3, 0, −1.2, −1.0, and +1.1 represent the A weighting relative response at the indicated octave band center frequencies.

The first method, which is most accurate, utilizes the spectrum of the noise being attenuated, and applies the formula

$$R = L_A - 10 \log S \qquad \textit{Eq. (7-1)}$$

where: R = dBA-reduction factor

L_A = workplace dBA noise level

$S = \text{antilog}\,[0.1 \times (L_1 - Q_1)] + \text{antilog}\,[0.1 \times (L_2 - Q_2)] + \text{antilog}\,[0.1 \times (L_3 - Q_3)] + \text{antilog}\,[0.1 \times (L_4 - Q_4)] + \text{antilog}\,[0.1 \times (L_5 - Q_5)] + \text{antilog}\,[0.1 \times (L_6 - Q_6)] + \text{antilog}\,[0.1 \times (L_7 - Q_7)]$

L_1, L_2, L_3, L_4, L_5, L_6, and L_7 denote octave band sound levels at 125, 250, 500, 1000, 2000, 4000, and 8000 Hz, respectively

Q_1, Q_2, Q_3, Q_4, Q_5, Q_6, and Q_7 account for the attenuation of a given hearing protector

The second method utilizes the difference between the dBC and dBA levels, and incorporates an adjustment of −3 dB to account for spectrum uncertainty. This method applies the equation

$$R = R_C - \delta \qquad \textit{Eq. (7-2)}$$

$$= 5.5 - 10 \log T - \delta \qquad \textit{Eq. (7-3)}$$

where: R = dBA-reduction factor

$R_C = 5.5 - 10 \log T$

$\delta = L_C - L_A$

L_C = workplace dBC noise level

L_A = workplace dBA noise level

$T = \text{antilog}\,(-0.1 \times Q_1) + \text{antilog}\,(-0.1 \times Q_2) + \text{antilog}\,(-0.1 \times Q_3) + \text{antilog}\,(-0.1 \times Q_4) + \text{antilog}\,(-0.1 \times Q_5) + \text{antilog}\,(-0.1 \times Q_6) + \text{antilog}\,(-0.1 \times Q_7)$

The third method, which is least accurate, utilizes only the dBA value of the noise environment, and incorporates a −8.5 dB adjustment to account for spectrum uncertainty. This method applies the formula

$$R = -1.5 - 10 \log T \qquad \textit{Eq. (7-4)}$$

where R and T are as defined for Equations 7-2 and 7-3.

SELECTION GUIDELINES

The selection of specific types of devices generally depends on:

a. Performance
b. Comfort
c. Application
d. Appearance
e. Cost

Both insert and muff-type protectors have distinct advantages and disadvantages. Some of the features of each type are listed in Table 7-1.[4]

COST

A 1975 NIOSH survey[5] studied the costs of three basic types of ear protectors. Costs were found to vary greatly among the companies surveyed depending upon the quantity of the purchase and any contract agreements between the company and the supplier. Average cost and range of prices were as follows:

	Average Cost	*Range*
Ear Plugs	\$0.61/pr.	\$0.35 – 0.93
Ear Muffs	\$6.12/pr.	\$3.40 –12.85
Individually Molded	\$5.50/pr.	Insufficient data

ISSUANCE AND FITTING

Hearing protective devices should be issued by an experienced nurse or technician who instructs the employee on proper wearing and cleaning. The devices should be individually fitted, and alternate types should be offered if the employee experiences a comfort problem.

Ear canals vary in size. Most manufacturers provide insert-type ear protectors in several sizes; however, no standards currently exist with regard to sizing. Typically, the following distribution of hearing protection sizes will be required for a typical work population:

Table 7-1. Comparison of Insert and Muff Type Hearing Protective Devices[4]

INSERT TYPE PROTECTORS

Advantages

1. They are small and are carried easily.
2. They can be worn conveniently and effectively with other personally worn items such as glasses, headgear, or hair styles.
3. They are relatively comfortable to wear in hot environments.
4. They are convenient to wear where the head must be maneuvered in close quarters.
5. The cost of sized earplugs is significantly less than muffs; however, hand-formed and personally molded protectors may be as much or more than muffs.

Disadvantages

1. Sized and molded insert protectors require more time and effort for fitting than for muffs.
2. The amount of protection provided by a good earplug is generally less and more variable between wearers than that provided by a good muff protector.
3. Dirt may be inserted into the ear canal if an earplug is removed and reinserted with dirty hands.
4. Earplugs are difficult to see in the ear from a distance; hence, it is difficult to monitor groups wearing these devices.
5. Earplugs can be worn only in healthy ear canals and, even in some healthy canals, a period of time is necessary for acceptance.

MUFF TYPE PROTECTORS

Advantages

1. The protection provided by a good muff-type protector is generally greater and less variable between wearers than that of good earplugs.
2. A single size of earmuffs fits a large percentage of heads.
3. The relatively large muff size can be seen readily at a distance; thus the wearing of these protectors is easily monitored.
4. Muffs are usually accepted more readily at the beginning of a hearing conservation program than earplugs.
5. Muffs can be worn even with many minor ear infections.
6. Muffs are not misplaced or lost as easily as are earplugs.

Disadvantages

1. Muffs are uncomfortable in hot environments.
2. Muffs are not as easily carried nor stored as earplugs.
3. Muffs are not as compatible with other personally worn items such as glasses and headgear as are earplugs.
4. Muff suspension forces may be reduced by usage, or by deliberate bending, so that the protection provided may be substantially less than expected.
5. The relatively large muff size may not be acceptable when the head must be maneuvered in close quarters.
6. Muffs are more expensive than most insert-type protectors.

Extra Small	5% of employees
Small	15% of employees
Medium	35% of employees
Large	30% of employees
Extra Large	15% of employees

The wearer's ear should also be inspected by an experienced technician or nurse to detect signs of infection or other disorders. The wearing of ear plugs can irritate an ear infection. If ear plugs are kept clean, however, they will ***not*** cause an ear infection.

ENFORCEMENT OF WEARING

Two types of programs may be implemented to encourage employees to wear their issued hearing protection:

a. *positive incentive program*
b. *negative incentive program*

A positive incentive program involves educating plant employees on the merits and benefits of wearing the hearing protection. The incentive program could include competition between departments. For example, a reward may be given to the department which has the best record of properly worn protectors.

A negative incentive program entails issuance of the protection on a mandatory basis. Employees who fail to wear the devices are given penalties, which may include verbal warnings, written warnings, suspensions, and severance of employment.

A NIOSH study[5] found that disciplinary actions for not wearing ear protectors were generally the same as standard procedures used in the overall safety program (e.g., for the habitual "forgetting" of hard hats or eye protectors). Examples of disciplinary programs used in six industries are listed in Table 7-2.

COMMUNICATION WITH HEARING PROTECTION DEVICES

A reluctance of workers to wear hearing protection is often due to the misconception that such devices will diminish their

Table 7-2. Six Companies' Programs of Disciplinary Action for Not Wearing Hearing Protection[5]

1	2	3	4	5	6
Oral Warning	Call to Employee's Attention	Two Verbal Warnings	Verbal Warning	Supervisor Report to Union	Verbal Warning
Letter in Personnel Folder	Notify Foreman of Infraction	Formal Written Warnings	Written Warning if within Six Months of No. 1	Union Responsible for any Disciplinary Action	Formal Letter in Personnel File
Two-Day Suspension	Verbal Warning	Transfer or Termination	Three-Day Suspension if within Six Months of No. 2		Letter to Safety Supervisor
Five-Day Suspension	Written Warning in Personnel Folder	Written Warning in Personnel Folder	Five-Day Suspension if within Six Months of No. 3		Termination of Employment
Ten-Day Suspension			Discharge if within Six Months of No. 4		

ability to hear. This notion has been proven to be false. Two studies[6,7] have indicated that wearing a conventional set of ear plugs or ear muffs where sound levels are approximately 90 dB in octave bands, or 97 dBA for flat spectra, should not interfere with, and may improve speech intelligibility for normal-hearing ears. With background noises below 85 dBA, intelligibility is generally the highest without protection. Figures 7-5 and 7-6 show the degree of speech intelligibility for normal ears with and without hearing protective devices and with high- and low-background noise levels.

Supporting these studies, at the 1977 9th International Congress on Acoustics, Wilkins and Martin concluded that there appears to be no basis for believing that hearing protective devices will diminish detection of warning signals.

FIELD ATTENUATION

One of the current shifts in professional opinion relates to the acceptance of the fact that hearing protective devices provide less attenuation when worn in the industrial environment than would be indicated by laboratory test data. In a paper presented at the 9th International Congress on Acoustics, Whittle and Robinson indicated that attenuation values should be reduced by 4 to 7 dBA for ear muffs and 8 to 11 dB for ear plugs because of wearer variability.

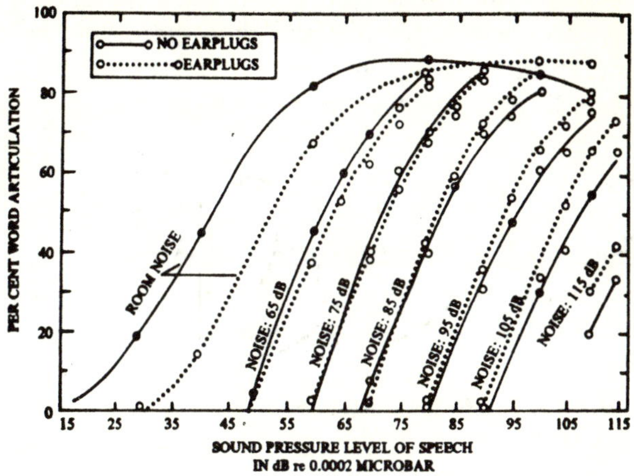

Fig. 7-5. The relationship between articulation and speech level with noise level as the parameter[6]

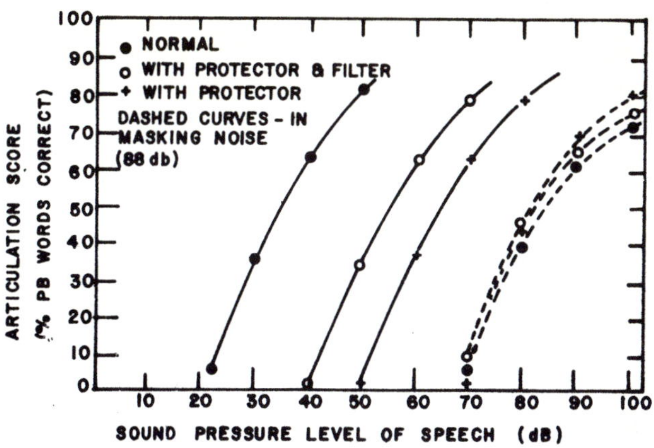

Fig. 7-6. Articulation curves, with and without hearing protection, in quiet and masking environments[7]

A NIOSH study, presented at a hearing on labeling of hearing protective devices, confirmed that there was significantly less attenuation achieved in tests in six Kentucky plants than would be indicated by laboratory test data.

ADEQUACY

Despite the fact that field attenuation may be significantly less than laboratory values, it must be recognized that very large attenuation values are often not necessary to provide adequate protection. Frank E. Wilcher, Jr., Executive Director of the Industrial Safety Equipment Association, has presented the following noise exposure profile of the American workforce exposed to more than 85 dBA:

Without Hearing Protectors	*Noise Level at the Ear*
.04%	110–115 dBA
.6	105–110
2.2	100–105
5.8	95–100
10.8	90–95
15.1	85–90

With a 15 dBA Noise Reduction Hearing Protector	*Noise Level at Ear*
.04%	95–100 dBA
.6	90–95
2.2	85–90

With a 20 dBA Noise Reduction Hearing Protector	*Noise Level at Ear*
.04%	90–95 dBA
.6	85–90

OSHA COMPLIANCE

Despite the encouragement of various industrial groups to allow the use of hearing protective devices as a permanent compliance measure, OSHA has held firm in allowing hearing conservation only as an interim measure while feasible engineering controls are being developed. One reason for this position, according to Dr. Morton Corn, former Assistant Labor Secretary, is that OSHA is geared to affect the conditions of the workplace through permanent improvements in the work environment.

EPA LABELING

The most significant federal activity related to hearing protective devices is the EPA labeling program. On 22 June 1977, EPA published in the *Federal Register* a program to require manufacturers to place noise labels on a wide range of products. These actions are designed to implement Section 8 of the Noise Control Act of 1972. "The newly proposed labeling program will permit informed consumer decisions by making possible comparisons of products related to noise or noise reducing characteristics," said EPA Administrator Douglas M. Costle. "As an example, the first product that EPA proposes for labeling is hearing protectors. In this case the label will bear a number between 0 and 31. The higher the number, the greater the product's effectiveness in excluding noise from a person's ear."

REFERENCES

1. Nixon, C. W., "Industrial Hearing Conservation," *Audiology & Hearing Education,* 33-41, April/May 1976.
2. Kroes, P.; Fleming, R.; and Lempert, B., "List of Personal Hearing Protectors and Attenuation Data," U.S. Department of Health, Education and Welfare Publication No. (NIOSH) 76-120, September 1975.
3. Webster, John C., "Updating and Interpreting the Speech Interference Level (SIL)," *J. Audio Engrg. Soc.*, 18:114, 1970.
4. "Industrial Noise Manual," American Industrial Hygiene Association, Third Edition, 1975.
5. Schmidek, M. E.; Layne, M. A.; Lempert, B. L.; and Fleming, R. M., "Survey of Hearing Conservation Programs in Industry," U.S. Department of Health, Education and Welfare Publication No. (NIOSH) 75-178, 1975.

6. Kryter, K. D., "Effects of Ear Protective Devices on the Intelligibility of Speech in Noise," *J. Acoust. Soc. Am.*, 18:413, 1946.
7. Michael, P. L., "Ear Protectors–Their Usefulness and Limitations," *Arch. Environ. Health*, 10:612, 1965.

8

The Measurement of Sound

To assess potential noise hazards, it is necessary to perform accurate acoustical measurements which may be compared with the various criteria for noise exposure. Excellent instrumentation has been available for several years which allows the investigator to perform virtually any type of noise measurement he may require with very reasonable accuracy. In the development of an industrial noise measurement program, the hearing conservationist must take care in selecting measurement instrumentation and procedures to insure that the data which is obtained is accurate and sufficient to provide the information required.

HEARING CONSERVATION AND OSHA REQUIREMENTS

The OSHA regulations clearly define sound environments which require corrective procedures in terms of A-weighted sound levels and employee exposure times. Recognizing sound levels which exceed these criteria is relatively simple, and generally requires only brief measurements. For the sole purpose of ascertaining that legal noise control obligations exist, it is generally unimportant to perform measurements of extreme accuracy. For example, it may not be relevant to distinguish between a noise dose of 180% and one of 250%, since both clearly exceed the OSHA guidelines. Acoustical measurements beyond simple dBA sound level readings are generally not necessary solely for the purpose of establishing legal compliance. Only for the case where legal compliance is marginal (i.e., sound levels very near 90 dBA or noise doses near 100%) would detailed sound level or exposure time data be appropriate. Also, where actual exposure time is not evident, such as in the case of intermittent noise sources, detailed dosimeter or time study measurements should be performed.

ENGINEERING DESIGN REQUIREMENTS

The development of engineering recommendations and designs requires advanced measurements. These include, at a minimum, octave-band sound-pressure level measurements, and often vibration analysis or narrow-band frequency analysis. Specific requirements will vary with the type of noise problem encountered. A technical description of acoustical instrumentation and measurement procedures is presented in the following sections of this chapter.

SOUND LEVEL METERS

A sound level meter consists of a microphone, electronic amplifier, filters, and a readout meter. These instruments are usually equipped to measure A-, B-, and C-Weighted sound levels, and are portable. Some are equipped with octave-band filters. A schematic of a typical sound level meter is shown in Figure 8-1. Several commercially available sound level meters are presented in Figure 8-2.

Microphones used for sound level meters are of three types: condenser, electret, and ceramic. The features of these types as they relate to specific measurement requirements are summarized in Table 8-1.

One of the primary differences between various sound level meters is accuracy. The American National Standard Specification for Sound Level Meters (ANSI S1.4-1971) sets the design-center response and three levels of accuracy for sound level meters. These accuracy levels are:

Type 1 – Precision

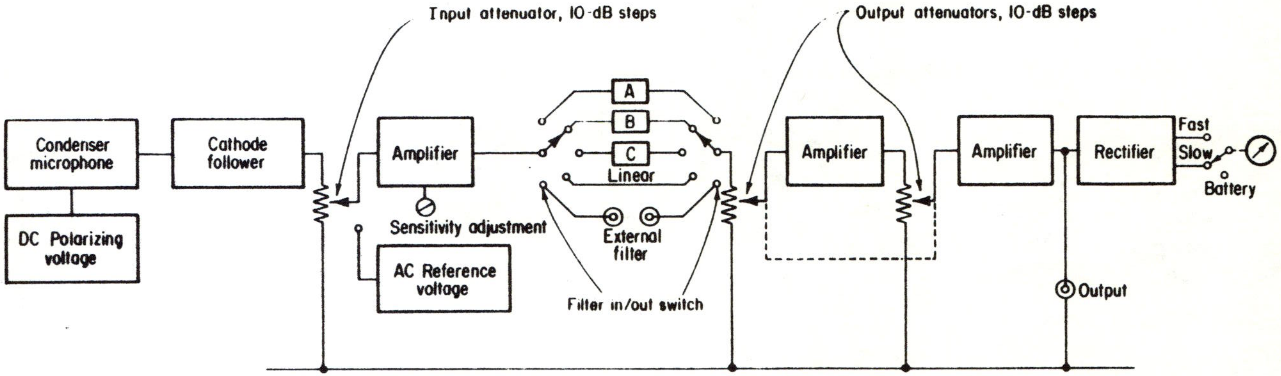

Fig. 8-1. Schematic representation of typical sound level meter. *(Courtesy of B&K Instruments, Inc.)*

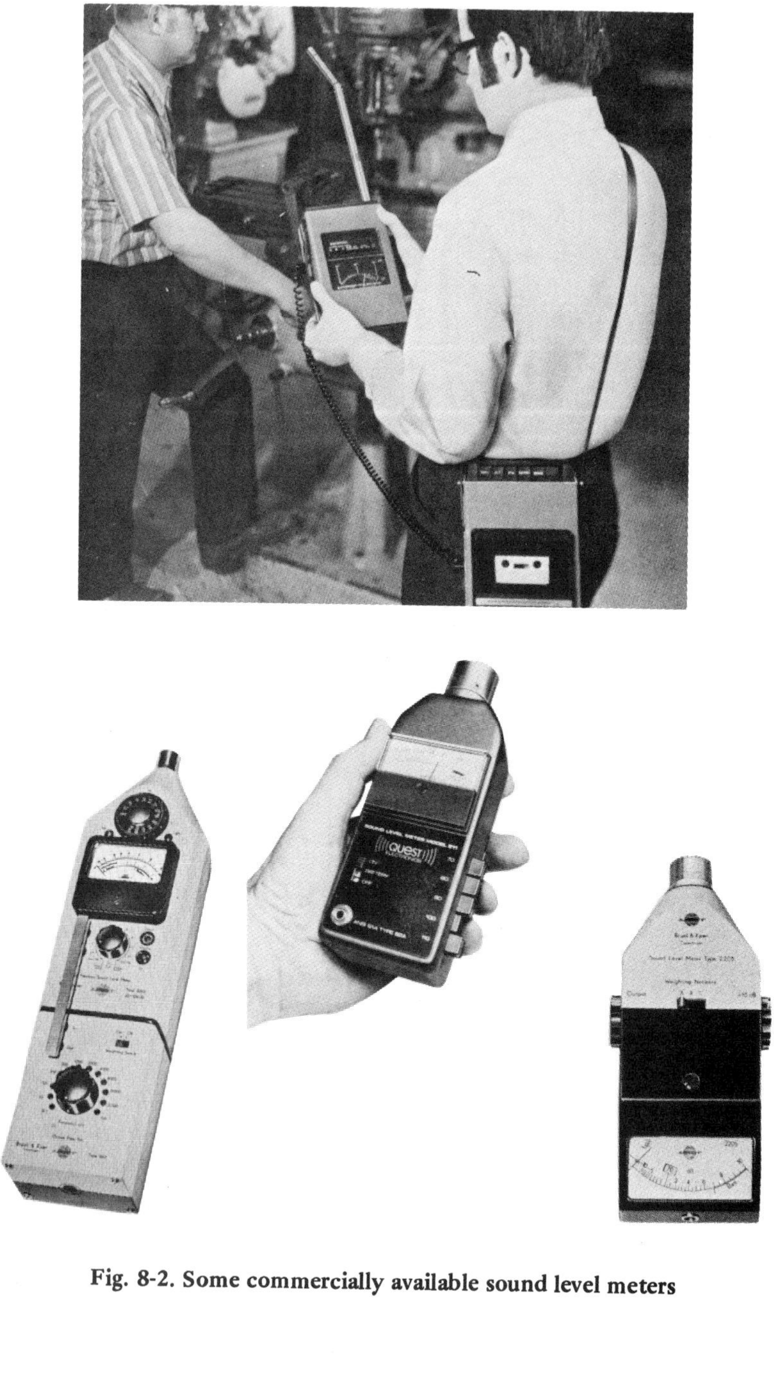

Fig. 8-2. Some commercially available sound level meters

Table 8-1. Importance of Performance and Environmental Factors for Various Microphone Applications[1]

	Microphone Characteristics	Microphone Application: Severe Field Use	General Field Use	Precision Field Use	Laboratory Use	Laboratory Standard Use
Performance Characteristics	Sensitivity	—	—	•	•	•
	Frequency Response	•	•	■	■	■
	Directional Response	•	•	■	■	■
	Dynamic Range	•	•	■	•	•
	Long-Term Stability	—	—	•	•	■
	Impedance	■	•	•	—	—
	Low-Frequency Response	—	—	•	•	•
	Mechanical Factors	—	—	•	■	■
Environmental Factors	Temperature Characteristics	•	•	•	•	•
	Humidity Characteristics	■	•	•	•	•
	Sensitivity to Vibration	•	•	•	—	—
	Corrosive Elements	■	•	•	—	—
	Cost	■	■	•	•	—
	Best Microphone Choice	Ceramic or Electret Condenser	Ceramic or Electret Condenser	Electret Condenser or Air Condenser	Electret Condenser or Air Condenser	Air Condenser

KEY:
- ■ Most Important Characteristics
- • Important Characteristics
- — Less Important Characteristics

Type 2 — General Purpose

Type 3 — Survey

The tolerance limits for the measurement of the A-Weighted Sound Level at random incidence are presented in Table 8-2.

The U.S. Department of Labor has recommended that a Type 1 or 2 be used for OSHA noise surveys. A Type 1 should be used for measurements where precise results are required.

OCTAVE-BAND FILTERS

In Chapter 1, an octave band was defined as a frequency range with a ratio of 2:1 between its high and low frequencies. Octave-band filter sets are commercially available, and some units are incorporated into sound-level meters. This instrument separates the noise spectrum into frequency bands by the use of

Table 8-2. Tolerance Limits for A-Weighted Response of a Sound Level Meter at Random Incidence, as Specified by ANSI S1.4-1971

Frequency (Hz)	*Type 1*	*Type 2*	*Type 3*
10	±4.0	—	—
12.5	±3.5	—	—
16	±3.0	—	—
20	±2.5	+5.0, −∞	+6.0, −∞
25	±2.0	+4.0, −4.5	+5.0, −6.0
31.5	±1.5	+3.5, −4.0	+4.5, −5.0
40	±1.5	+3.0, −3.5	+4.0, −4.5
50	±1.0	±3.0	±4.0
63	±1.0	±3.0	±4.0
80	±1.0	±3.0	±3.5
100	±1.0	±2.5	±3.5
125	±1.0	±2.5	±3.0
160	±1.0	±2.5	±3.0
200	±1.0	±2.5	±3.0
250	±1.0	±2.5	±3.0
315	±1.0	±2.0	±3.0
400	±1.0	±2.0	±3.0
500	±1.0	±2.0	±3.0
630	±1.0	±2.0	±3.0
800	±1.0	±1.5	±3.0
1,000	±1.0	±2.0	±3.0
1,250	±1.0	±2.0	±3.0
1,600	±1.0	±2.5	±3.5
2,000	±1.0	±3.0	±4.0
2,500	±1.0	+4.0, −3.5	±4.5
3,150	±1.0	+5.0, −4.0	±5.0
4,000	±1.0	+5.5, −4.5	±5.5
5,000	+1.5, −2	+6.0, −5.0	±6.5
6,300	+1.5, −2	+6.5, −5.5	±7.0
8,000	+1.5, −3	+6.5, −6.5	±7.5
10,000	+2.0, −4	+6.5, −∞	+7.5, −∞
12,500	+3.0, −6	—	—
16,000	+3.0, −∞	—	—
20,000	+3.0, −∞	—	—

electronic filters. While an ideal filter would have a perfect cut-off at the low- and high-frequency limits of an octave band, real filters feature a rolloff, as shown in Figure 8-3.

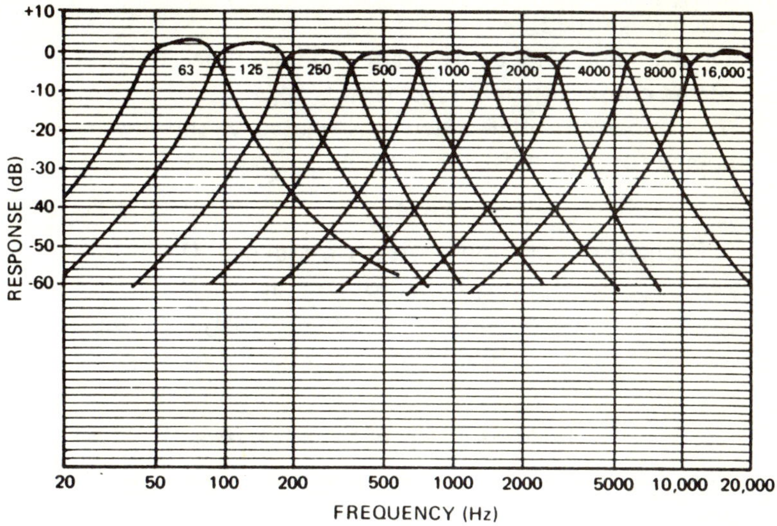

Fig. 8-3. Frequency response for an octave-band filter

Octave-band filters are generally used for basic engineering design. By observing the frequency in which the maximum sound pressure levels occur, system characteristics which may relate to the noise generation may be identified and corrected.

FREQUENCY ANALYZERS

For general requirements, the measurement of dBA, dBC, and octave-band sound pressure level values should be adequate. More information may be required to diagnose the noise of a machine. Analyzers are used to determine the exact frequency characteristics of a machine and to correlate its overall noise to specific noise-generating mechanisms. These instruments are generally not portable, but are designed for laboratory analysis. Analyzers are specified as two types:

1. Constant bandwidth analyzers
2. Constant percentage analyzers

A constant bandwidth analyzer has a bandwidth which is independent of frequency. A constant percentage analyzer has a bandwidth which is always a fixed percentage of the frequency to which it is tuned.

Octave band, 1/3 octave band, and 1/10 octave band filters are of the constant percentage band type.

The upper cut-off frequency is related to the lower cut-off frequency for acoustical analyzers by:

$$f_u = K\ f_l \qquad \textit{Eq. (8-1)}$$

where: f_u = Upper cut-off frequency, Hz
f_l = Lower cut-off frequency, Hz
K = Constant relating to analyzer type, as indicated in Table 8-3.

Table 8-3. Values of K for Analyzers

Analyzer	*K*
Octave Band	2
1/2 Octave Band	$\sqrt{2}$ = 1.414
1/3 Octave Band	$\sqrt[3]{2}$ = 1.26
n-th Octave Band	$\sqrt[n]{2}$

The geometric mean frequency of an analyzer is given by:

$$f_o = \sqrt{f_l f_u} \qquad \textit{Eq. (8-2)}$$

where: f_o = Geometric mean frequency, Hz
f_l = Lower cut-off frequency, Hz
f_u = Upper cut-off frequency, Hz

The bandwidth, BW, (in Hertz), of an analyzer is expressed as:

$$BW = f_u - f_l \qquad \textit{Eq. (8-3)}$$

For a constant percentage band analyzer it is:

$$BW = \frac{f_u - f_l}{f_o} \times 100\% \qquad \textit{Eq. (8-4)}$$

The bandwidth increases with frequency for a constant percentage filter. Figure 8-4 shows the bandwidth as a function of frequency for constant percentage and constant frequency bandwidth filters. As seen in the figure, a constant frequency filter is not always narrower than a constant percentage filter. When a full octave is being measured, more sound energy is being received by the analyzer than if only a one-third octave band was admitted to the analyzer. As illustrated in Figure 8-5, the relative sound pressure levels are less for the one-third octave band spectrum. Care should be taken in reviewing published noise data with regard to the analyzer type being used for the measurement. When comparing a one-third octave band graph with an octave band presentation, the one-third octave band values must be combined to obtain the equivalent octave band sound pressure levels.

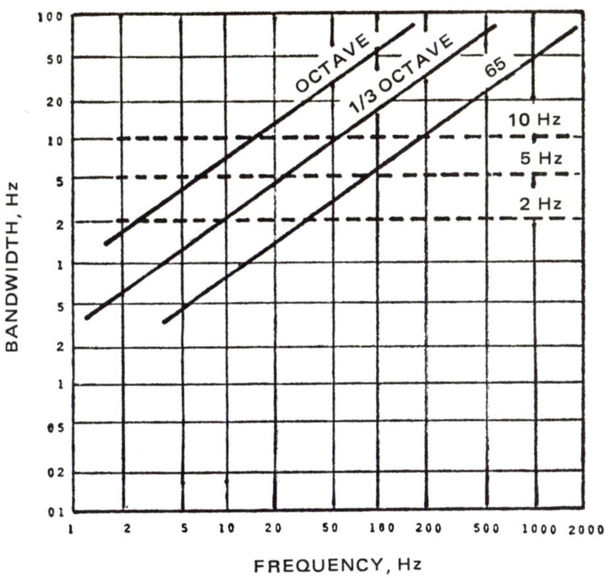

Fig. 8-4. Bandwidth vs. frequency for constant percentage and constant frequency filters[1]

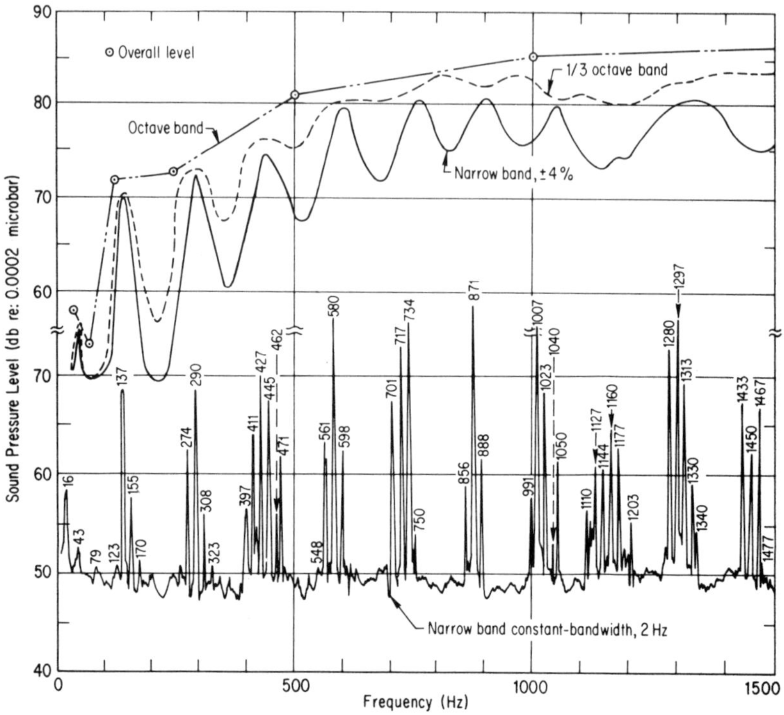

Fig. 8-5. Comparison of acoustical data sample analyzed with octave band, one-third octave band, and narrow band filters[3]

The sweep rate of an analyzer is the speed which the analyzer can electronically scan the frequency spectrum. The transient response of a filter to abrupt spectrum changes imposes a sweep rate limitation on filters, given approximately by:

$$SR = \frac{BW^2}{8} \qquad Eq. (8\text{-}5)$$

where: SR = Sweep rate, Hz/sec
BW = Bandwidth, Hz

Thus, there is a trade-off between time of analysis and information obtained in the use of filters. The consultant must design his analysis around each specific application. Often a noise spectrum may be studied first by one-third octave band analysis, and a narrow band analyzer can then be used to study the problem frequency areas.

CALIBRATION

To verify the accuracy of acoustical measurements, it is necessary that the instrumentation be calibrated. There are two types of calibration which must be performed: laboratory calibration and field calibration.

Laboratory calibration is performed by the original equipment manufacturer or an acoustical laboratory using reciprocity or electrostatic techniques. This type of calibration should be performed annually. For greatest reliability, the calibration should be traceable to the National Bureau of Standards.

Prior to, and after each set of sound level readings, the measurement system should be field calibrated. This is achieved by the use of an accurate sound source which introduces a reference sound level into the microphone. The procedure involves placing the calibrator over the microphone and adjusting a sound level meter calibration knob until the meter reading corresponds to the reference sound pressure level. A field calibration set-up is shown in Figure 8-6.

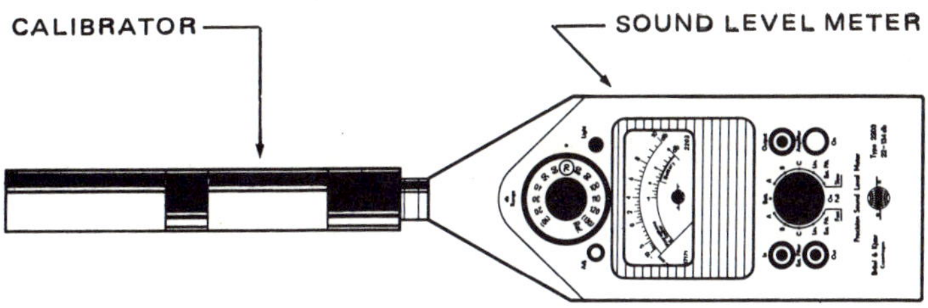

Fig. 8-6. Field calibration of a sound level meter using a pistonphone type calibrator
(Courtesy of B & K Instruments)

MEASUREMENT PROCEDURES

For accurate measurement of employee noise exposure, the sound level meter should be placed six inches to one foot from the operator's ear position. Care should be taken to insure that all equipment and noise sources are operating in a normal manner when measurements are performed.

The key to operating a sound level meter is to use it in a manner which will not alter the sound field being measured. This includes:

1. Hold the meter away from the operator's body to prevent sound reflections. Also, the operator must not be located between the meter and the noise source. The effect of an observer on a measurement is shown in Figure 8-7.

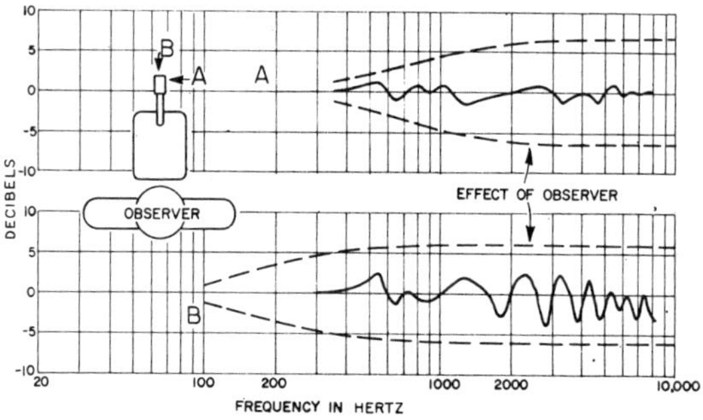

Fig. 8-7. The effect on frequency response due to the presence of an observer

2. Perform the measurement away from any other objects which may block or reflect the sound.
3. Orient the microphone as recommended by the manufacturer. The proper way to hold a sound level meter fitted with a random-incidence calibrated microphone is shown in Figure 8-8. The response for curves for various angles of incidence are shown in Figure 8-9.

Background noise can cause errors in acoustical measurements whenever it is within 10 dB of the noise being measured. Measurements should be performed with the noise source off.

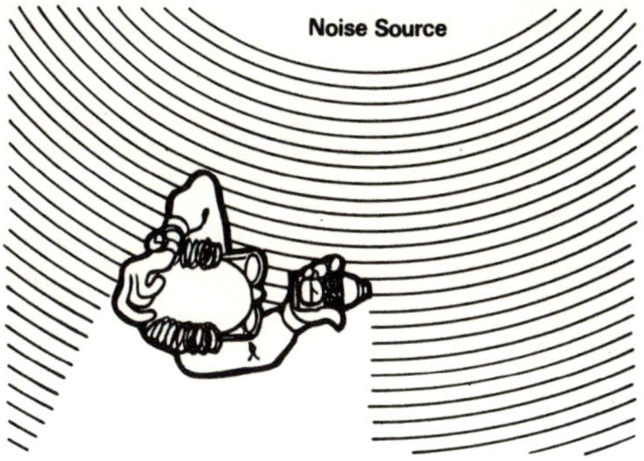

Fig. 8-8. The proper manner to hold a sound level metter fitted with a random-incidence calibrated microphone *(Courtesy of GenRad)*

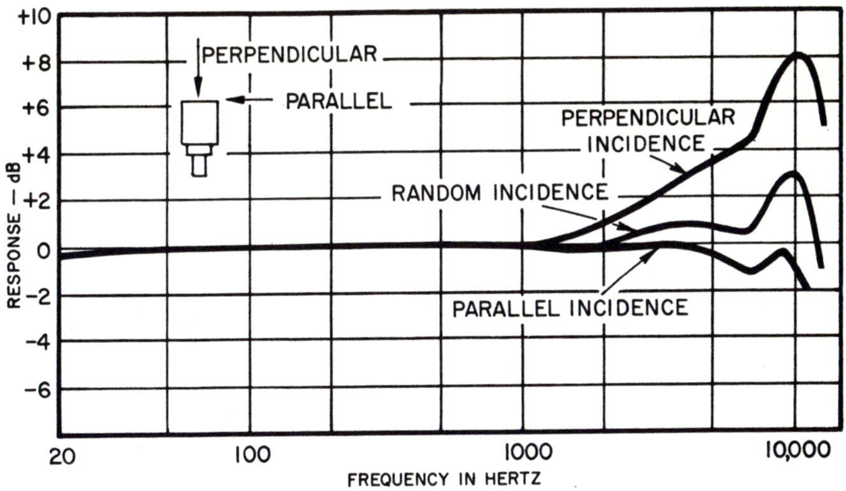

Fig. 8-9. Typical response curves for ceramic microphone *(Courtesy of GenRad)*

If the difference is less than 10 dB, the correction factors of Table 8-4 should be subtracted from the measured noise source level to account for background noise.

Table 8-4. Correction Factors for Background Noise

Difference Between Total Noise and Background Noise, dB	*Level to Be Subtracted from Total Noise, dB*
3	3
3.5	2.5
4	2
5 – 6	1.5
6 – 8	1.0
8 – 10	0.5

MEASURING NOISE WHICH VARIES

Since the OSHA regulation relates to employee exposures to noise rather than to a noise level per se, noise surveys must accurately describe two parameters:

1. Sound levels in dBA
2. Employee exposure time, hours

The daily noise exposure of an employee is described by:

$$D = \frac{C_1}{T_1} + \frac{C_2}{T_2} + \dots\dots\dots\dots + \frac{C_n}{T_n} \qquad \textit{Eq. (8-6)}$$

where: D = daily noise dose
C_n = time of actual exposure to a sound level, hours
T_n = allowable time of exposure to noise, as specified by OSHA regulation, hours (see Table 1-1)

Noise dose values may be translated to equivalent A-Weighted (dBA) sound levels by reference to Table 8-5.

The daily noise dose must be calculated or measured within a reasonable accuracy not only to assess compliance with the OSHA guidelines, but also to establish design goals for required noise reductions. For steady-state noise environments with continuous employee exposure, determination of an accurate daily noise dose may be quite simple: Determination of accurate noise doses for environments where sound levels and/or employee work routines vary, however, may be exceedingly difficult.

Table 8-5. Equivalent A-Weighted Sound Level and Noise Dose Values

dBA	*Noise Dose, %*	*dBA*	*Noise Dose, %*
85	50	100	400
86	57	101	462
87	66	102	526
88	76	103	606
89	87	104	696
90	100	105	800
91	115	106	920
92	131	107	1040
93	152	108	1194
94	174	109	1404
95	200	110	1600
96	230	111	1860
97	264	112	2105
98	283	113	2424
99	355	114	2857
		115	3200

DOSIMETERS

One method for the determination of noise doses is the use of dosimeters. Dosimeters are integrating sound meters which are worn by employees as they perform their normal work routine. These units are worn for a fixed time period, usually eight hours, and read out directly in noise dose values. A typical dosimeter is shown in Figure 8-10.

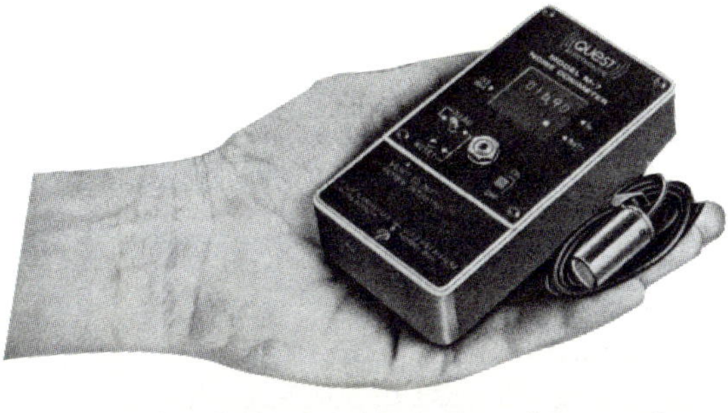

Fig. 8-10. A noise dosimeter *(Courtesy of Quest Electronics)*

Research has been conducted by the Mining Enforcement and Safety Administration (MESA) to determine the optimum location on the body for the wearing of a dosimeter. In the case of a free field,[4] the optimum position was found to be "on top of the subject's shoulder, oriented parallel to the body axis." In the case of a reverberant field,[5] the optimum location was found to be "the left breast pocket with a 90° orientation." The optimum position for a semireverberant field was found to be at the top of the left shoulder with a 90° orientation.

There is currently no standard governing the accuracy of dosimeters; however, the American National Standards Institute (ANSI) is in the process of developing such a standard. In lieu of a specific standard, manufacturers often apply ANSI S1.4-1971 criteria to establish the accuracy of the instrument. While this assessment is not incorrect, it should be recognized that it only assesses the frequency response characteristics of the instrument. The effect of errors in dosimeter response, as measured in decibels, may be translated to noise doses by use of Table 8-6.

Dosimeter accuracy is highly dependent upon proper wearing by the employee. For proper measurement, the wearer should be instructed as follows:[7]

1. Wear the dosimeter for a full 8-hour shift.
2. Let the person conducting the survey remove, turn off, and read out the dosimeter.
3. Do not whistle or talk into the microphone.
4. Leave the microphone in the position that it is originally placed.
5. Do not place the dosimeter on any machinery or motors, or remove the unit during the lunch break.

A list of the features of various commercially available dosimeters is presented in Table 8-7.

CALCULATING NOISE DOSE VALUES

As an alternative to the measurement of noise exposures using dosimeters, noise dose values may be calculated from A-Weighted sound level data, as measured with a conventional meter, and exposure time information.

Table 8-6. The Effect of dB Error on % OSHAct Exposure Measure[6]

dB Error	% OSHAct Reading when Expecting 100%	dB Error	% OSHAct Reading when Expecting 100%
+ 6.5	246.2	− .1	98.6
+ 6.0	229.7	− .2	97.3
+ 5.5	214.4	− .3	95.9
+ 5.0	200.0	− .4	94.6
+ 4.5	186.6	− .5	93.3
+ 4.0	174.1	− .6	92.0
+ 3.5	162.4	− .7	90.8
+ 3.0	151.6	− .8	89.5
+ 2.5	141.4	− .9	88.3
+ 2.0	132.0	− 1.0	87.1
+ 1.5	123.1	− 1.5	81.2
+ 1.0	114.9	− 2.0	75.8
+ .9	113.3	− 2.5	70.7
+ .8	111.7	− 3.0	66.0
+ .7	110.2	− 3.5	61.6
+ .6	108.7	− 4.0	57.4
+ .5	107.2	− 4.5	53.6
+ .4	105.7	− 5.0	50.0
+ .3	104.2	− 5.5	46.7
+ .2	102.8	− 6.0	43.5
+ .1	101.4	− 6.5	40.6
0	100.0		

In calculating employee noise doses, a rigid approach utilizing production records and time-and-motion studies would be ideal. If such data have not already been compiled for industrial engineering analysis or other purposes, however, the acquisition of such data solely for noise exposure definition would be unnecessarily difficult and costly. The application of statistical sampling of noise exposures is more practical and may provide very accurate results.

In any physical measurement where repeated observations of a statistically controlled sample are made, fluctuations in the measured variable are usually found. Where these variables are random, statistical methods may be applied to present the noise measurements. The arithmetic mean is used as the measure of central tendency of the measured distribution, and the standard deviation is the measure of dispersion. Calculated confidence limits measure the degree of certainty of the calculated mean.

Table 8-7. A Comparison of Audio Noise Dosimeters[8]

Manufacturer	Dosimeter/ Monitor Model No.	Readout Model No.	Type of Dosimeter	Calibrator No.	Field Calibration Adjustment to Dosimeter	Microphone Type	Microphone Integral or Remote	Readout Capa-bility, %	Threshold dB	Exchange Rate, dB	A-Weighting Standard	Battery Power (Monitor)
Bendix	ADS-3000-1	ADS-3000-2	Monitor	Built Into Readout	Yes	Ceramic	Remote	99,999	80-90	3,4,5	ANSI Type II	1 9-volt Battery
Bruel & Kjaer	4425	—	Self-Contained	B&K 4230	Yes	B&K 4125 Condenser Microphone	Both	9999	90	5	ANSI Type II	2 9-volt Batteries
Bruel & Kjaer	4424	—	Self-Contained	B&K 4230	Yes	B&K 4125 Condenser Microphone	Both	9999	80	3	International Standards Organization	2 9-volt Batteries
Columbia	SPL-105	—	Self-Contained	Columbia SPL-10D	Yes	Ceramic Microphone	Remote	199.9	80/85	5	ANSI Type II	1 9-volt Battery
Du Pont	D-100	R-150 or R-225	Monitor-Readout	Du Pont C-114	No, Return to Manufacturer	Shure 99A401B Ceramic Micropone	Remote	3,200	90	5	ANSI Type II	1 9-volt Battery
Du Pont	D-285	R-150 or R-225	Monitor-Readout	Du Pont C-114	No, Return to Manufacturer	Shure 99A401B Ceramic Microphone	Remote	3,200	85	5	ANSI Type II	1 9-volt Battery
Du Pont	D-376	R-150 or R-225	Monitor-Readout	Du Pont C-114	No, Return to Manufacturer	Shure 99A401B Ceramic Microphone	Remote	3,200	90/85	5	ANSI Type II	1 9-volt Battery
GenRad	1954-9710	1954-9720	Monitor-Readout	Built Into Readout	Yes	Ceramic Microphone	Both	999.9	80-90	3,4,5	ANSI Type II	1 9-volt Alkaline Battery
MSA	85	—	Self-Contained	MSA 695182	Yes	Electret	Remote	9999	85	5	ANSI Type II	1 9-volt Battery
MSA	90	—	Self-Contained	MSA 695182	Yes	Electret	Remote	9999	90	5	ANSI Type II	1 9-volt Battery
Quest	M-7	—	Self-Contained	Quest CA-12	Yes	Ceramic Microphone	Remote	999.99	90	5	ANSI Type II	1 9-volt Alkaline Battery
Simpson	891	—	Self-Contained	Simpson No. 887	Yes	Electret	Remote	9999	90	5	ANSI Type II	1 9-volt Battery
Tracoustics	ND-100	ND-100C	Monitor-Readout	Built Into Readout	No, Return to Manufacturer	Ceramic Microphone	Remote	999.9	90/85	5	ANSI Type II	Rechargeable NICAD Batteries

The arithmetic mean, X, is simply the arithmetic average of a set of individual measurements, and is given by:

$$\overline{X} = \frac{\Sigma X}{N} \qquad \textit{Eq. (8-7)}$$

where: $\overline{X}$ = Arithmetic mean
N = Total number of measurements in the set

The standard deviation, $\hat{\sigma}$, is the root mean square of the deviations from the mean and is given as:

$$\hat{\sigma} = \sqrt{\frac{\Sigma (X - X)^2}{N - 1}} \qquad \textit{Eq. (8-8)}$$

The 90 percent confidence limit is the limit within which the arithmetic mean may be expected to occur nine times in ten in a series of measurement samples. The confidence limit is equal to the standard deviation times a constant ($a\hat{\sigma}$). The constant, a, is dependent upon the number of measurements made. Table 8-8 gives the values of a.

Variations in employee noise exposure may be either temporal or spacial in nature. These may be due to two factors:

1. Variations in the noise source intensity
2. Variations in the employees work.

When employees at a fixed work location are engaged in various work operations, or if noise sources within an area vary, it is necessary to define the temporal characteristics of the workspace. Once the percentage of time that each noise event occurs is defined, the sound level associated with each event may be measured and the daily noise dose may be calculated. This may be accomplished by selecting random time periods on various days and sampling work activities during these periods. During each random period, the investigator should select a strategy for identifying an employee's work activity at selected time increments (typically every 5 seconds) for a given time period. The results of each time period should be compiled into percentage values for each activity. The mean, standard deviation and confidence limit values should then be calculated from the percentage values associated with the activities defined for each time period.

Table 8-8. Factor "a" for Calculating % Confidence Limits ($\bar{x} \pm a\hat{\sigma}$)

Sample Size N	*90% Confidence Limit "a" Value*	*95% Confidence Limit "a" Value*
2	4.50	9.00
3	1.70	2.50
4	1.15	1.59
5	.93	1.23
6	.81	1.04
7	.73	.93
8	.63	.83
9	.62	.76
10	.59	.72
11	.55	.69
12	.52	.63
13	.49	.60
14	.48	.58
15	.45	.55
16	.44	.53
17	.42	.51
18	.40	.49
19	.39	.48
20	.38	.47
21	.37	.45
22	.36	.44
23	.35	.42
24	.34	.42
25	.34	.41
26	.33	.40
27	.32	.39
28	.32	.38
29	.31	.37
30	.30	.36
40	.26	.31
60	.21	.25
120	.15	.18
N Greater than 120	$\frac{1.645}{\sqrt{N}}$	$\frac{1.96}{\sqrt{N}}$

As an example of temporal sampling, application in a foundry cleaning area will be reviewed. Eight employees in a work area were involved in the intermittent use of six types of tools: pneumatic chipping hammers, pencil grinders, straight grinders, disc grinders, hammers and hoists. Three noise abatement measures were proposed:

1. Acoustical curtains to isolate chipping noise from adjacent workers;
2. Exhaust silencers on pneumatic disc grinders;
3. Exhaust mufflers on hoists.

To assess the reduction in the overall employee noise doses due to these measures, it was necessary to model the noise exposure components of the workspace. This eas accomplished by randomly selecting four time periods during the workday when operations would be considered "typical." During each period, activities of employees were observed at five-second intervals for a period of 20 minutes. The observation tallies were converted to percentage values and are shown in Table 8-9. An encouraging verification of the sampling technique was found when the results of a time and motion study were within 3% of results obtained by statistical sampling for a grinding operation. Mean, standard deviation, and confidence limit values were calculated from the time period percentage values. As shown in Table 8-10 the average percentage values were converted to exposure times associated with an eight-hour work day. Based on measured sound levels associated with each operation and these time estimates, the noise dose was calculated to be 807%. Dosimeter measurements by an OSHA compliance officer indicated readings of 803% and 804%. Utilizing predicted sound levels which would be expected due to the abatement measures, a new noise dose of 623% was calculated.

SPATIAL SAMPLING[9]

Spatial average sound level values are of interest in situations where employees move about in a workspace. Typical examples would be supervisors and maintenance and inspection personnel. In these situations where an employee's location may be anywhere in the workspace at any point in time, the employee's average daily noise dose may be approximated from the mean sound level of the workspace and his average daily time spent in that area.

Table 8-9. Summary of Percent of Time Cleaning Operators Are Engaged in Various Activities

Activity	*Sample 1*	*Sample 2*	*Sample 3*	*Sample 4*	*Average*	σ	*90% C.L.*
Chipping	20	20	22	35	24	6	7
Pencil Grinder	4	7	3	0	4	3	3
Straight Grinder	6	0	0	7	3	3	4
Disc Grinder	37	28	37	25	32	6	6
Hammering	0	0	0	4	1	2	2
Hoist	0	5	2	2	2	2	2
No Source	33	40	36	27	34	5	6

Note: Percentages based on four statistical samples of work activity observations.

Table 8-10. Calculated Noise Doses for Cleaning Operators

Operation	*Dominant Noise*	*Time, Hours*	*Sound Level, dBA*	*Noise Dose*	*Level with Abatement*	*New Dose*
Chipping	chipping	1.8	112	4.5	112	4.5
Disc Grinder	grinder	1.8	203	1.38	95	0.45
	adjacent chipping	0.6	105	0.6	100	0.3
Pencil Grinder	grinder	0.3	95	0.8	95	0.8
	adjacent chipping	0.1	105	0.1	100	0.05
Straight Grinder	grinder	0.2	100	0.1	100	0.1
Hammering	hammering	0.1	100	0.5	100	0.5
Hoist	hoist	0.2	102	0.13	93	0.4
No Source	adjacent chipping	0.6	105	0.6	100	0.3
	far chipping	0.6	98	0.21	93	0.11
	ambient	1.3	95	0.32	93	0.25
				8.07		6.23

Another situation where the mean sound level may be of interest would be in assessing the influence of various noise abatement measures on the overall noise of a workspace. For example, in a rail car manufacturing facility, a noise abatement program included expanding a workspace to minimize crowded work conditions and to silence several ventilation fans. To identify the noise reduction effectiveness of these measures, the sound levels of the workspace were randomly sampled and documented as 94.4 dBA±, .95 (90% confidence limit). This value would serve as a baseline for comparison with the mean environmental level after the modifications were effected.

The most statistically proper method of random spatial sampling is to place a square grid overlay onto a workspace floorplan and to number each grid intersection. Points are then randomly selected to identify measurement locations. The mean, standard deviation, and confidence limit values are then calculated from the measured data. A disadvantage of this method is that some random measurement points may be superimposed on items of equipment or at locations which employees would not be expected to frequent. This problem may be remedied by discarding these inappropriate locations and selecting additional random points as measurement locations. The exact number of locations to be selected is dependent upon the accuracy desired.

A second technique which may be applied to spatial sampling is to identify a walking path throughout a workspace, and to perform sound level measurements at fixed intervals (typically every 5–10 feet) along the path. Either a random path may be selected, or a path which would be most descriptive of actual employee work routines may be selected. While the selection of periodic measurement points along a predetermined path destroys the random nature of the sampling, it may be recognized that this technique may accurately describe actual employee noise exposure. Also, since there may be no correlation between noise source intensities and worker mobility patterns, it would typically be found that sound level data points will assume a distribution which is reasonably Gaussian. Thus, concepts of mean, standard deviation, and confidence limits may be loosely applied, even though the results will be only "pseudo-random."

To insure that significant errors are not encountered in noise survey results, it is advisable that both dosimeter and calculated noise dose values be obtained. If a significant discrepancy is encountered, the source of error should be investigated.

TAPE RECORDERS

Magnetic tape recorders are used to store acoustical data for remote analysis. This may include either a frequency spectrum analysis or for making subjective comparisons. Recorders would seldom be used for simple noise surveys, however they may be necessary for more sophisticated analysis.

The magnetic tape recorder should be selected with a frequency response at least equal to the ANSI specifications for the sound level meter being used. When using tape recording analysis, the entire system should be calibrated, from microphone to data reduction equipment.

REFERENCES

1. Kundert, Warren R., "Everything You've Wanted to Know About Measurement Microphones," *Sound and Vibration,* 12, 3:10-23, March 1978.
2. Courtesy of Bruel & Kjaer, Cleveland, Ohio.
3. Mitchell, L. D. and Lynch, G. A., "Origins of Noise," *Machine Design,* May 1969.
4. Marraccini, L. C., "Optimum Microphone Placement for the Personal Noise Dosimeter," *NOISEXPO 1974 Proceedings,* 184-187.
5. Muldoon, T. L., "Response Variations of a Microphone Worn on the Human Body," Report of Investigation 7810, U.S. Bureau of Mines.
6. Conn, D. O., "The Audio Dosimeter," *National Safety News,* October 1972.
7. Seiler, J. P., "Noise Dosimeters," *Sound and Vibration,* 18-22, March 1977.
8. Seiler, J. P., "Noise Dosimeter Update," *Sound and Vibration,* 32-33, March 1978.
9. Miller, R. K., "Statistical Sampling of In-plant Noise Environments," presented at Noisexpo 78, 23 March 1978.

9

Engineering Control of Noise

Today's engineer assigned with the task of reducing in-plant noise levels is fortunate that the technology already exists to solve most of industry's noise problems. Prior to the passage of the Occupational Safety and Health Act of 1970, noise control was a mysterious science to most engineers. With the current interest in noise abatement, however, the engineer has available a wealth of information to which he may refer to assist in solving noise problems. Literally dozens of "tests" and hundreds of articles and papers have been published on the subject. Over eighty colleges and universities offer courses on noise control and acoustics. Although a few types of noise problems remain unsolved (such as certain riveting operations, some chemical milling operations, certain grinding operations, oxygen lances, rock drills, and weaving looms), most types of machinery have been quieted. In many cases tried and proven noise reduction systems may be installed in lieu of undertaking an extensive design program. In many cases a noise control program requires only purchasing new, quieter equipment.

The principles of noise control are most easily understood when the noise system is broken into its various elements. All noise systems may be viewed as consisting of three components:

1. Source
2. Path
3. Receiver

NOISE GENERATION

All noise sources generate noise by one of the two following mechanisms:

1. Acoustical radiation from a vibrating surface.
2. Aerodynamic turbulence.

VIBRATION RADIATION

Sound may be produced by the movement of a vibrating structure which, in turn, sets into motion the air molecules which are coupled to it.

Prediction of vibration and noise for any mechanical system is both complex, and specific to each system's parameters. Specifically, one must consider (a) vibration energy, and (b) system response.

The vibrational energy may be computed from the basic equations of dynamics. Impact forces may be computed from:

$$K.E. = \tfrac{1}{2}mv^2 \qquad \textit{Eq. (9-1)}$$

where: K.E. = kinetic energy at impact
m = mass
v = velocity

and

$$F = ma \qquad \textit{Eq. (9-2)}$$

where: F = impact force
a = deceleration of impact

Momentum transfer during impact must consider elasticity. Conservation of momentum is given by:

$$m_1 v_1 + m_2 v_2 = m_1 v_1' + m_2 v_2' \qquad \textit{Eq. (9-3)}$$

System response is dependent upon the following parameters:

1. Vibrational response
   a. mass
   b. stiffness
   c. damping

2. Acoustical radiation efficiency
   a. surface area
   b. critical coincidence frequency

The vibrational response of a system is generally a maximum at its resonant frequency, given by:

$$f_r = \frac{1}{2\pi}\sqrt{\frac{k}{m}} \qquad \textit{Eq. (9-4)}$$

where: f_r = resonance frequency
k = stiffness
m = mass

Centrifugal forces are proportional to the mass imbalance

$$F = m\,e\,\omega^2 \qquad \textit{Eq. (9-5)}$$

where: m = equivalent eccentric mass
e = eccentricity
ω = rotational velocity

The frequency of this force is:

$$f = \text{rpm} \div 60 \qquad \textit{Eq. (9-6)}$$

Other vibrational force analysis may be determined by basic conservation of energy or momentum equations.

Higher resonant frequencies may occur at integer multiples of this frequency due to nonlinearities, and at noninteger multiples due to higher order modes of vibration.

Maximum sound levels generally occur in any system at either the frequency of vibration energy or system resonant frequency. In noise reduction, the frequency of maximum acoustical energy should be identified. If this frequency is a system resonant mode, vibration damping may be an appropriate solution. If the frequency corresponds to a forcing function, system response alterations would generally be of little consequence.

In assessing the acoustical radiation efficiency of a structure, it should be recognized that acoustical energy is generally directly proportional to the radiation surface area. Each mechanical system will have an acoustical critical coincidence frequency, where the speed of sound in the structure equals the speed of sound in air. This frequency may be computed for steel from the relationship:

$$f_c = \frac{500}{t} \qquad \textit{Eq. (9-7)}$$

where: t = thickness, inches

The structure will be an efficient radiator of sound at and above this frequency. Below this frequency, the structure will be a less efficient radiator of sound.

The (theoretical) near field sound pressure level above the coincidence frequency of a structure may be computed from the measured or predicted vibration levels by the following relationship:

$$L_p = L_v - 20 \log f + 150 \qquad \textit{Eq. (9-8)}$$

where: L_v = vibration level re 1 g
L_p = sound pressure level in dB
f = frequency

Below the coincidence frequency, the part sound radiation will be 3-4 dBA/octave less than predicted by the equation. The equation is valid only for frequencies with wavelengths less than the panel dimension.

AIR NOISE

The generation of air noise results from the creation of fluctuating pressures due to turbulence and shearing stresses as high velocity gas interacts with the ambient air or solid surfaces. Radiating sources called "eddies" are formed with the high frequency noise being generated in the mixing shearing region and the lower frequency noise being generated downstream in the region of large-scale turbulence (see Figure 9-1).

Theoretically, as the pressure ratio between reservoir (line pressure) and ambient air is increased, the velocity of the air at the discharge nozzle increases. However, when a pressure ratio of approximately 1.9 is reached, the flow velocity through the

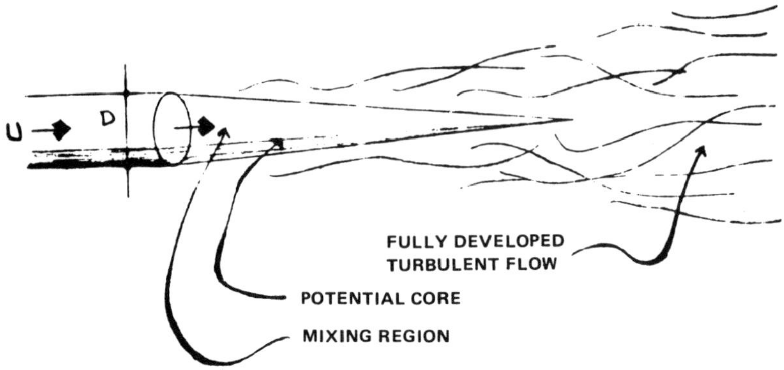

Fig. 9-1. The sound created by air leaving a jet is due to density fluctuations in the air flow. It is in the turbulent field of the jet flow that these density fluctuations occur and sound is created.

nozzle becomes sonic, i.e., reaches the speed of sound, and further increases in reservoir pressure do not significantly increase the flow velocity. When this critical pressure ratio of 1.9 is reached, the nozzle is said to be "choked." It may be assumed, however, that at 80-100 psi, the air jets are generally in a condition of choked flow.

Based on the work of Lighthill, the overall sound power from a subsonic or sonic jet can be calculated from:

$$P = \frac{K\rho A v^8}{c^5} \qquad \textit{Eq. (9-9)}$$

where: A = area of jet nozzle
ρ = density of ambient air
v = jet flow velocity
c = speed of sound
K = constant of proportionality

It is clear that the velocity of the gas stream has the greatest influence on jet noise. Cutting the velocity in half would lower the sound power by 24 decibels. However, halving the area would account for a decrease of only 3 decibels. For practical calculation of jet noise, Equation (9-9) may be modified to the following form:

$$P = \frac{eM^5 \rho V^3 A}{2} \qquad \textit{Eq. (9-10)}$$

where: V = average flow velocity through nozzle
M = Mach number of flow (V/c)
ρ = density of ambient air
A = nozzle area
e = constant of proportionality of the order of 10^{-4}

For choked flow (Mach 1) conditions, the factor eM^5 is approximately 3×10^{-5}.

The sound power from Equation (9-10) may be converted to decibels utilizing the relationship:

$$L_W = 10 \log \frac{P}{10^{-12}} \qquad \textit{Eq. (9-11)}$$

The frequency of peak noise level can be calculated to the first order from the following equation:

$$f_o = \frac{SV}{D} \qquad \textit{Eq. (9-12)}$$

where: S = Strouhal number (a constant) = 0.2 approximately for a wide range of conditions
V = nozzle exit velocity
D = nozzle diameter

NOISE CONTROL

Three approaches to noise control should be considered for any noise problem:

1. The noise *source* may be modified.
2. Noise may be blocked or reduced along the *path* from the source to the receiver.
3. Sound may be isolated from the *receiver* by means of barriers, operator location, or hearing protection.

Six types of noise control systems may be considered to solve any noise problem:

1. Sound barriers
2. Sound absorbers
3. Vibration damping
4. Vibration isolation

5. Mufflers and silencers
6. Machine redesign, process modification, or noise source elimination

BARRIERS

The most fundamental approach to noise reduction is to interpose a wall between the sound source and receiver. The wall may take the form of:

1. an enclosure of the noise source (machine),
2. the enclosure of the receiver (employee), or
3. a barrier between the two.

The noise reduction, or difference between the sound levels on either side of the wall, will vary depending upon which of these constructions is employed; however, the physical acoustical properties of the wall is the key element in the calculation of the noise reduction for all three of these designs.

The basic characteristic used to describe the acoustical performance of a wall is the transmission loss. The transmission loss, abbreviated TL, is defined as 10 times the logarithm (base 10) of the incident sound energy on a wall to the sound transmitted through it, or:

$$TL = 10 \log_{10} \frac{w_i}{w_t} \qquad \textit{Eq. (9-13)}$$

where: TL = transmission loss, dB
w_i = incident sound energy, watts
w_t = transmitted sound energy, watts

The Sound Transmission Class, STC, is a single numerical average of a barrier's transmission loss performance, and is used for preliminary acoustical assessments.

Flexible curtains of mass-loaded vinyl have excellent sound transmission loss properties and may be used to block airborne sound. Typical applications include:

- Complete or partial machine enclosures
- Movable walls to isolate noisy machine areas from other quieter areas
- Localized enclosures for machine parts

Acoustical curtains are constructed of 0.5 to 1.0 psf lead-filled vinyl and may be installed with grommets or on sliding tracks. It is important that the curtains extend to the floor and be sealed at the edges with Velcro fasteners for maximum attenuation. Installation details of enclosure construction are given in Figure 9-2.

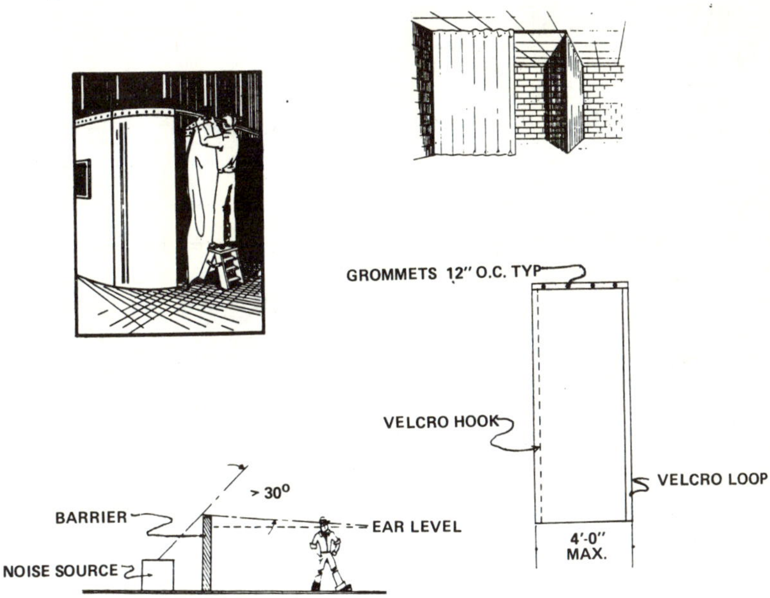

Fig. 9-2. Installation guidelines for acoustical curtains

SOUND ABSORPTION

The sound absorption coefficient, α, represents the ratio of the sound absorbed to the sound incident on any material, and varies from 0 to 1. An α value equal to 1 indicates that all of the incident acoustic energy is absorbed, while an α value equal to 0 means that all of the incident acoustic energy is reflected. Sound absorption values vary with frequency, and are dependent upon material thickness.

Whenever machinery is operated within enclosed spaces, sound levels will be increased to some extent due to reverberation. When this reverberant sound level increase becomes significant, it is appropriate to install sound absorptive materials on the ceiling above offending machinery. A simplified procedure can be used to estimate the increase in noise due to the reflected component, as shown in Figure 9-3.

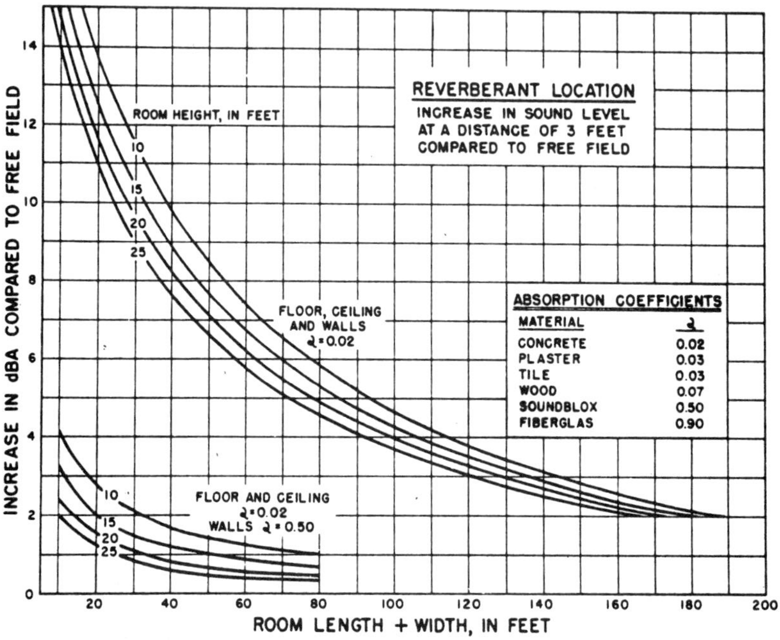

Fig. 9-3. Simplified procedure for estimating increase in noise due to reverberation

The most convenient method of employing sound absorption is the installation of acoustical baffles, as shown in Figure 9-4. Where large surface areas are to be treated, a spray-on treatment may be most economical.

Attention should also be given to machine location within a room. These relationships are shown in Figure 9-5.

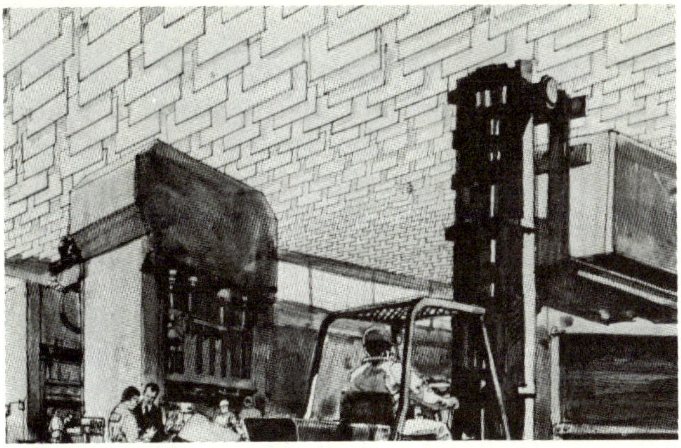

Fig. 9-4. Acoustical ceiling baffles *(Courtesy of United States Gypsum)*

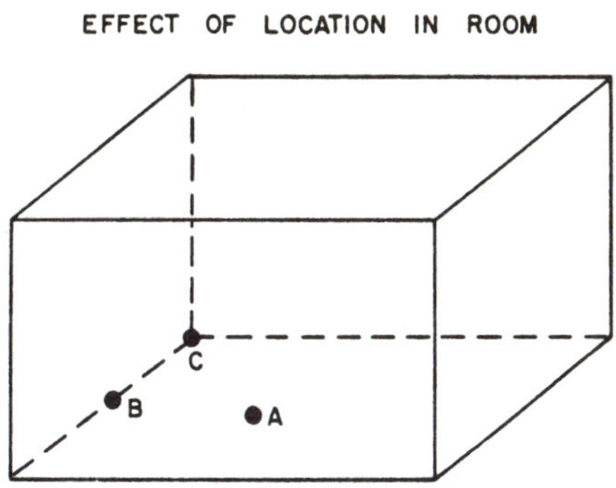

LOCATION	Q
A	2
B	4
C	8

Absorption Coefficient	Change Location	Increase In SPL
0.02	A to B	1.5
0.02	A to C	3.0
0.50	A to B	3.0
0.50	A to C	6.0

Fig. 9-5. Effect on location in room

VIBRATION DAMPING

Since the physical mechanism of most noise problems is acoustical radiation from vibrating structures, it is most logical to reduce noise by means of vibration damping. The term "damping" refers to the design property of materials which converts vibrational energy into heat energy.

Three measures are frequently used to qualitatively describe a material's damping characteristics:

1. Loss Factor, η
2. Decay Rate, Δ
3. Damping Factor, ξ

The loss factor, η, is the dimensionless damping-stiffness ratio of a viscoelastic material.

Another common measure of vibration damping is the decay rate, Δ, expressed in decibels per second, and is defined as the rate of natural attenuation for free vibrations within a material. The decay rate is related to the loss factor by the approximate relationship:

$$\Delta = 27.3\ \eta\ f \qquad \textit{Eq. (9-14)}$$

where: Δ = Decay rate, dB/sec
η = Loss factor (dimensionless)
f = Frequency, Hz

The damping factor, ξ, is defined as the ratio of material damping to critical damping:

$$\xi = C/C_c \qquad \textit{Eq. (9-15)}$$

The damping factor is related to the loss factor by the approximate relationship:

$$\xi = \eta/2 \qquad \textit{Eq. (9-16)}$$

Free layer damping, also referred to as extensional or surface damping, is the most commonly and easily applied. Damping treatment of this type may be a viscous substance which is applied similarly to an automobile undercoating, or may be in the form of a sheet or tile which is bonded to the structure being damped.

Constrained layer damping involves sandwiching a layer of viscoelastic material between the structure being damped and an outer constraining layer. This type of damping finds application where structural members are quite thick, or where a large vibration reduction is required.

VIBRATION ISOLATION

A basic way to control vibrationally-induced noise is to isolate the driving force of the machinery from the adjacent structure. Machinery which has a driving force frequency in the 10-60 Hz range and is rigidly mounted to a building foundation may easily create a very annoying environment for office workers. Vibration isolators will generally reduce this annoyance.

Vibration isolators may be of the spring type, rubber mount, or any other type, as illustrated in Figure 9-6.[1]

The steps for selecting spring-type vibration isolators are:[2]

1. Establish that part of the total weight that is on the footing in question.
2. Determine lowest forcing deflection required for degree of transmission percent required (see Table 9-1); 5% is normally adequate.
3. Choose a suitable isolator that will sustain the load and have the proper deflection. Isolator manufacturers often list spring constants (lb/in. deflection).
4. Ensure that deflection is uniform for each footing.
5. For more complex isolation problems, submit the data from vibration tests to isolator manufacturers for more exact specifications.

MUFFLERS AND SILENCERS

Silencers find application for the control of noise due to engines (internal combustion, diesel, etc.) and from high-velocity air flows. There are six basic types of silencers,[3] as shown in Figure 9-7. They are:

1. *Absorptive silencer.* This is the most common type of silencer, and takes the form of a duct lined on the interior with a sound absorptive material.

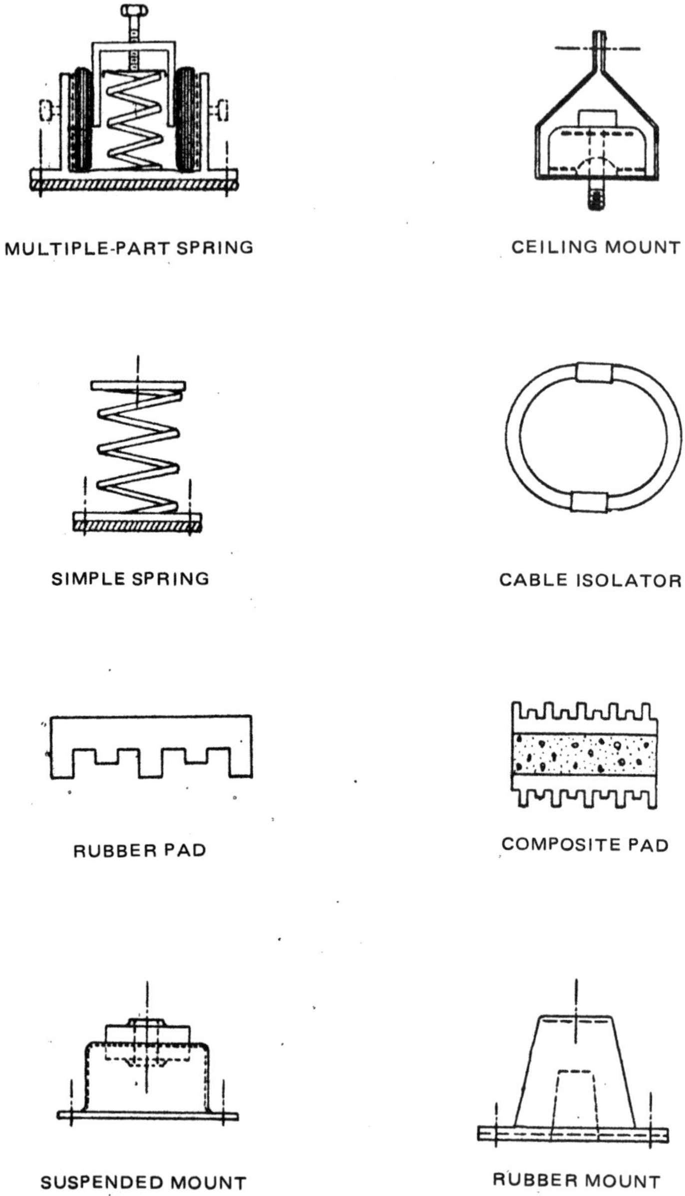

Fig. 9-6. Classification of vibration isolators[1]

Table 9-1. Required Static Deflection (Inches) for Common Industrial Speeds or Forcing Frequencies (Base is Assumed Immovable)[2]

Speed		Vibration Transmission (percent)				
rpm	freq.	0.5%	1.0%	5.0%	10%	25%
3600	60	0.55	0.27	0.06	0.03	0.01
2400	40	1.2	0.62	0.13	0.07	0.03
1800	30	2.2	1.1	0.27	0.12	0.05
1600	27	2.8	1.4	0.29	0.15	0.07
1400	23	3.6	1.8	0.38	0.20	0.09
1200	20	4.9	2.5	0.52	0.27	0.12
1000	17	7.1	3.6	0.74	0.39	0.18
800	13		5.6	1.2	0.61	0.28
600	10			2.1	1.1	0.49
400	7			4.6	2.4	1.1

2. *Reactive expansion chamber.* This type performs by reflecting sound energy back toward the source so as to cancel some of the oncoming sound energy.
3. *Reactive resonator.* This type functions in approximately the same way as the reactive expansion chamber type.
4. *Plenum chamber.* This device allows the sound to enter a small opening in the chamber; that sound which has not been absorbed by the chamber's acoustical lining leaves by a second small opening, generally at the opposite end of the chamber.
5. *Lined bend.* Sound energy flowing down a passage is forced to turn a corner, the walls of which are lined with acoustical material. The sound energy is thus forced to impinge directly on a sound-absorbing surface as it reflects its way around the corner; each successive impingement takes sound energy from the traveling wave.
6. *Diffuser.* This device doesn't actually reduce noise. In effect, it prevents the generation of noise by disrupting high-velocity gas streams.

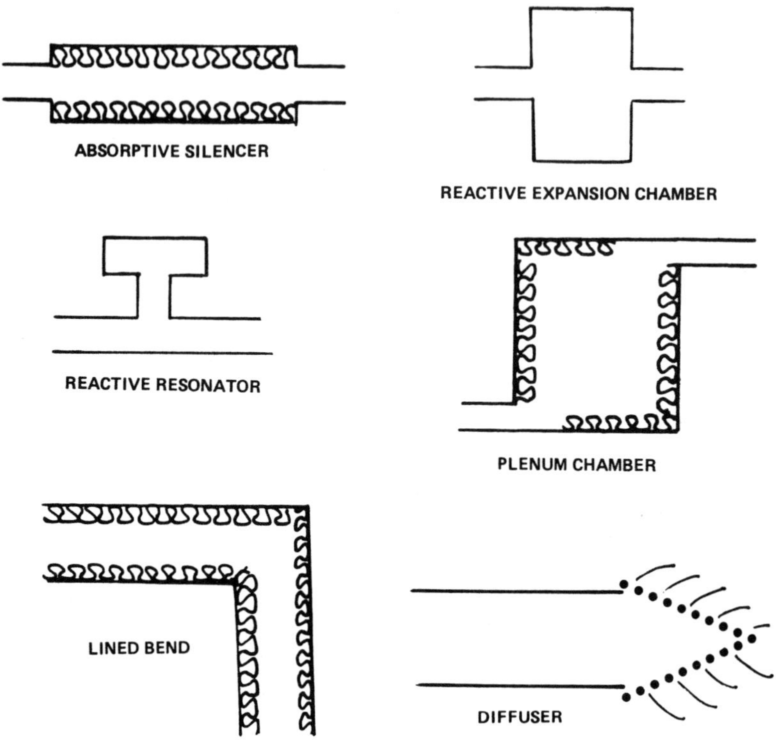

Fig. 9-7. Basic silencers[3]

SPECIFIC NOISE CONTROL SOLUTIONS

While the number of different types of machines which create industrial noise control problems are too numerous to cover in any single text, it is helpful to consider specific solutions to some of the more common types of industrial machinery. The following machines are covered in the following sections of this chapter: motors, ventilation fans, presses, saws, air exhausts, air leaks, vibrators, cutting operations, pneumatic tools, and gears.

MOTORS

With approximately two million motors sold a year, motor noise is of great concern. The two primary types of motor enclosures are the drip-proof (DRPR) and the totally enclosed, fan-cooled (TEFC) motors. the DRPR cools itself by pulling in outside air and circulating it around the electrical conductors, while the TEFC motor uses a fan to accomplish cooling. The high speed (3500 rpm and above) and TEFC motors are noisier than their slower speed and DRPR counterparts.

Solutions to motor noise problems include muting or muffling the inlet and outlet air and isolating or dampening the vibrations. Motors with horsepower ratings of 75 or more often require abatement. Motors below this rating do not normally generate noise levels that are above 90 dBA; however, these smaller motors may contribute to other equipment noise, and the additive levels may exceed 90 dBA.

Several motor manufacturers have developed new lines of quiet motors with higher horsepower ratings. This has been accomplished through quiet fan designs and minor internal modifications. To insure minimum motor noise levels, specifications that sound pressure levels are not to exceed 85 dBA at 3 feet and that sound power levels are not to exceed 95 dBA, should be made to manufacturers for any new motors purchased.

VENTILATION FANS[4,5]

Sound levels of fans are influenced by the following variables:

- Speed or rpm of the motor
- Velocity output of the fan
- Number of blades
- Blade shape and pitch
- Horsepower
- Diameter

The following fan laws relate to noise generation:

$$\text{CFM}_a = \text{CFM}_b \times \left(\frac{\text{size}_a}{\text{size}_b}\right)^3 \times \left(\frac{\text{RPM}_a}{\text{RPM}_b}\right)^1 \qquad \textit{Eq. (9-17)}$$

$$HP_a = HP_b \times \left(\frac{size_a}{size_b}\right)^5 \times \left(\frac{RPM_a}{RPM_b}\right)^3 \qquad Eq.\ (9\text{-}18)$$

$$SPL_a - SPL_b = 70 \log_{10}\left(\frac{size_a}{size_b}\right) + 50 \log_{10}\left(\frac{RPM_a}{RPM_b}\right) \qquad Eq.\ (9\text{-}19)$$

The sound levels due to the roof ventilation fans often exceed 85 dBA, and occasionally exceed 90 dBA. Silencing of these fans is frequently required to achieve satisfactory ambient levels in a plant. Three approaches may be considered:

1. *Fan Silencers.* The installation of silencers is considered the most effective abatement method. The "straight-through" type should be used so as to minimize air flow impedance. Commercially available systems generally cost about $2000 per unit. Installation costs may be twice the unit cost.
2. *Replacement Blades.* There are commercially available replacement blades of a multitude of configurations for noise reduction purposes that are compatible with most existing horsepowers, rpms and sizes.
3. *Hanging Barrier.* Suspending a barrier directly below the fan, obstructing the line-of-sight to the workfloor may be considered. If a sound absorptive barrier of twice the fan diameter were hung 1½ times the diameter below the unit, a noise reduction of 1-4 dBA may be expected. A more restrictive barrier may provide noise reductions up to 10 dBA; however, such units are generally impractical, because a 10 to 15 percent impedance of the fan's air flow would result.

When purchasing new fan units, the engineer should always include noise level specifications.

PRESSES

In terms of the work force exposed to press noise and the difficulty of silencing, presses probably could be ranked as the number one noise problem in the United States today.

In operations involving shearing, blanking and punching using punch presses, the large impact forces exerted by the descending punch on the plate placed upon the die and the shearing action take place simultaneously. A typical operation is illustrated schematically in Figure 9-8. A plate to be blanked is placed upon a stationary die and is engaged by a descending punch whose width is slightly less than the clearance between these spaced parts of the die. The portion of the plate between these spaced parts of the die is, thus, sheared from the body of the plate and moved downward ahead of the punch.[6]

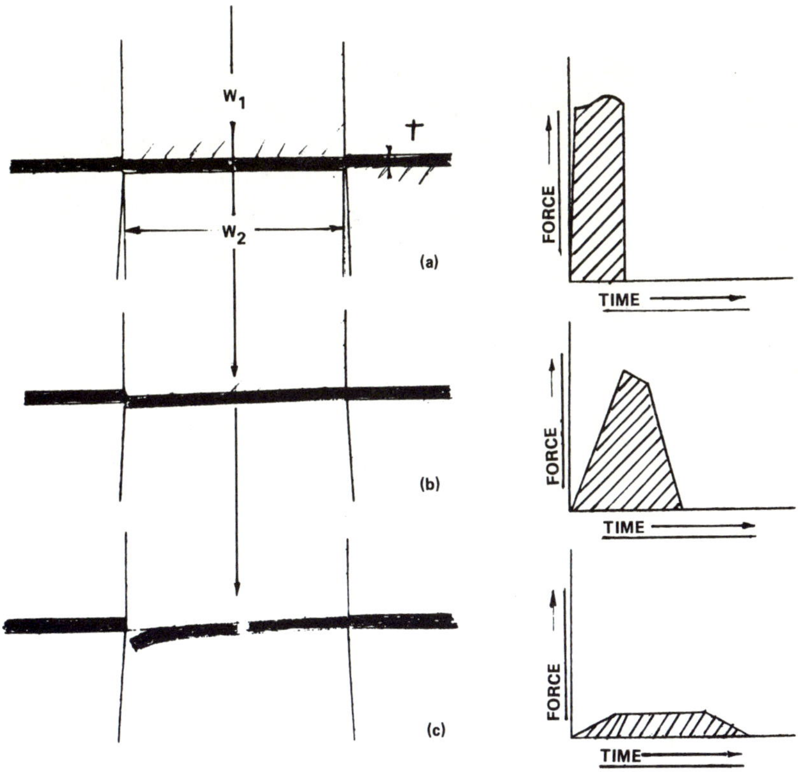

Fig. 9-8. Schematic illustration of blanking operation showing the effect of shear angle of the punch. The force-time diagram for each condition is shown at the right.[6]

If the punch is designed as illustrated in Figure 9-8 (a), all the shearing action occurs simultaneously. A large force is thus involved, as indicated by the height of the shaded area at the right of the figure. If the lower face of the punch is slightly inclined, as illustrated in Figure 9-8 (b), the shearing action is distributed over a greater part of the stroke. The maximum force then endures for a shorter period and the duration of the force is increased, as shown by the shape of the shaded area. A further increase in the angle of the lower face of the punch, as shown in Figure 9-8 (c), brings about a pronounced decrease in the duration of the force.[6]

In an operation involving the punching of several holes at one stroke of a press, a similar reduction of total force can be attained by stepped punches, as illustrated in Figure 9-9. The punching of successive holes occurs progressively, and not all the punches are operative at a given time. Where pierced blanks are required, punching and blanking operations frequently are performed in multistage dies. Perforations are first made in the material; the material is then moved the length of one stage and the piece is blanked around the perforations while first-stage operations are being performed on the following increment of material. It is desirable, where possible, to equalize the work between stages and to keep the strokes in the several stages out of phase to maintain the individual impulses as small as possible.[6]

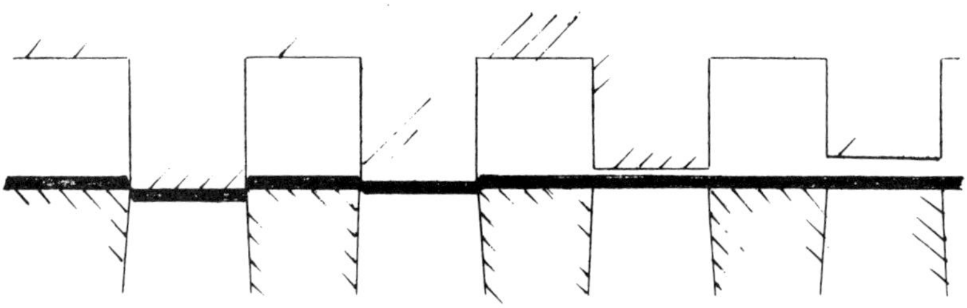

Fig. 9-9. Stepped punches for punching several holes at one stroke of a press[6]

While slanted or inclined dies and stepped punches are used in many plants, it should be pointed out that this is generally not a complete solution to noise control. Even with these die modifications, sound levels may be above 90 dBA. Also, such die modifications are not applicable to all parts.

The installation of acoustical enclosures to reduce press noise may also be considered. With the noise being radiated from the localized area of the die and plunger, a localized enclosure would provide significant noise reduction. Assuming the use of heavy materials and nearly airtight construction, a noise reduction of 10-15 dBA may be expected.

A partial enclosure of a press by Storment and Pelton[7] achieved a noise reduction from 108 dBA to 89 dBA. See Figure 9-10.

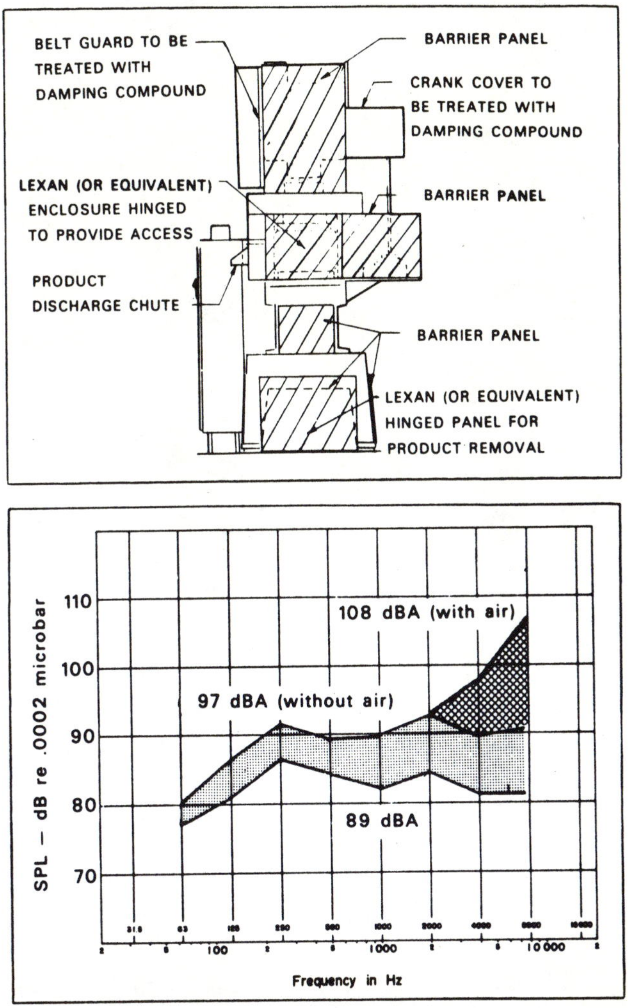

Fig. 9-10. Punch press partial enclosure and noise reduction achieved.[7]

SAWS

Noise from cut-off saws comes from two vibrating sources:

1. The saw blade.
2. The workpiece, which is usually largely unconstrained.

Since both the workpiece and blade are noise contributors, an acoustical enclosure is generally the best approach to noise control. One enclosure design[8] is shown in Figure 9-11.

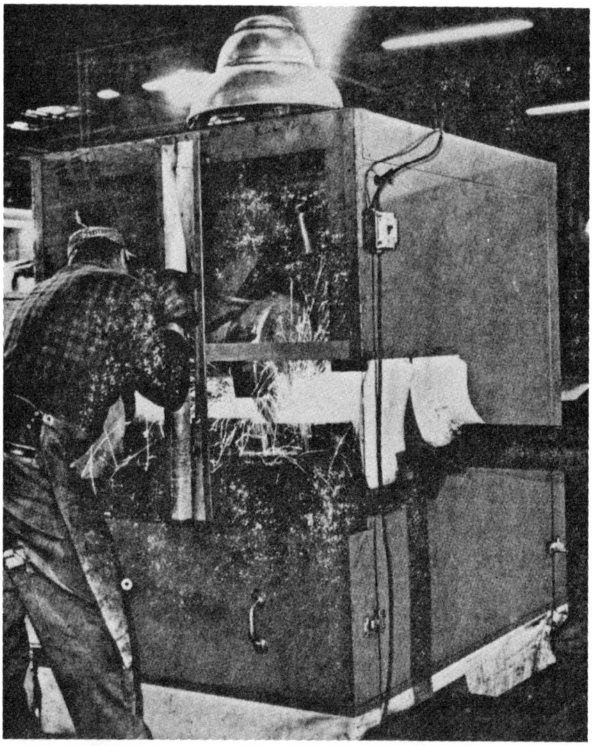

Fig. 9-11. Acoustical enclosure for metal cut-off saw operation.[8]

Workpieces pass transversely through slots in the enclosure. Flaps of lead-loaded vinyl close off the opening and reduce to a small amount the unavoidable leakage area when a workpiece is present. The front, above saw bed height, is closed by two doors whose surface is mostly ¼-inch clear plastic (polymethylmethacrylate). This plastic provides very good vision. The doors close with a gap the width of the control lever. Each door has a flap of lead-loaded vinyl about 3 inches wide to close the gap. The lever pushes aside the flaps only where it protrudes. Thus, the leakage toward the worker is greatly reduced. A 13 dBA noise reduction was achieved.

For operations involving the sawing of thin-walled parts, it may be possible to design damping fixtures to be applied to the part.

Where the noise generated by the workpiece can be reduced, the blade must be treated also. This may be accomplished by installing a large stiffening collar on the blade, extending as near the base of the teeth as allowable by the stock thickness (the collar must cover 30% of the blade to be effective). A layer of vibration damping material should be installed between the collar and blade.

As an alternative to the collar, the center portion of the blade not utilized for cutting may be treated with a constrained layer damping treatment. This treatment should cover as large an area as possible (30% is the minimum for effectiveness), and must not come into contact with the material being cut.

AIR EXHAUSTS

Sound levels generated by air exhaust, where concentrated air flow is not required, may be silenced by the installation of pneumatic mufflers which diffuse the air stream. The specification of an optimum pneumatic silencer for any application should be based upon:

- Sound level reduction
- Low pressure drop
- Durability
- Nonclogging features for the air contaminants present
- Economy

Mufflers should be periodically inspected for wear and effectiveness. If necessary an in-line filter system may be installed to prevent muffler clogging.

AIR LEAKS

Air leaks from pneumatic systems are often found to be major contributors to the overall noise in many plants. It is important that a program be implemented including an inspection and maintenance procedure, performed on a regular basis, to identify air leaks such as due to the following:

- Broken air hoses and cracked pipes
- Worn fittings and couplings
- Faulty valves
- Air-operated devices left on when not in use

It should also be noted that such a maintenance program would be a significant cost and energy conservation measure, as well as an important part of a noise abatement program. The air consumption and cost associated with air leakage from a sharp-edged orifice continuously at 100 psig with air at 7 cents per 1000 cubic feet is as follows:

Diameter of Opening, Inches	*Air Flow, cfm*	*Annual Cost of Waste (8 hour shifts)*	*Annual Cost (continuous)*
1/32	1.62	$ 14.19	$ 59.60
1/16	6.49	56.85	238.78
1/8	26.0	227.76	956.59
1/4	104.0	911.04	3826.37

VIBRATORS

Vibrators are frequently for conveying materials and parts. The following approaches to noise control may be considered:

1. Install mufflers on pneumatic vibrators.
2. Substitute electric vibrators for noisier pneumatic units.
3. Use "cushioned stroke" vibrators.
4. Investigate alternate means of material handling.
5. Regulate vibrator use such that it is on only when required.
6. Operate vibrator at minimum required capacity.
7. Partially dampen system being vibrated.

8. Redesign system being vibrated to eliminate any large surface areas which would be prime sound radiators.
9. Enclose vibrator.

CUTTING OPERATIONS

One recent study[9] found that the workpiece itself radiates most of the noise involved in cutting operations, especially where stainless steel and light metals are used. This noise may be reduced by loading the workpiece with damping plates, as shown in Figure 9-12. Only the free surfaces are used for damping the workpiece. The stiffness of the plates in combination with the loading used has to be adjusted to the stiffness of the workpiece. A typical damping plate construction is shown in Figure 9-13. Using this approach, a noise reduction from 108 dBA to 85 dBA was reported.

Tool chatter and also machining vibrations may often be reduced by the use of a lubricant or by modifying cutting parameters: cutting, speed, depth of cut, etc.

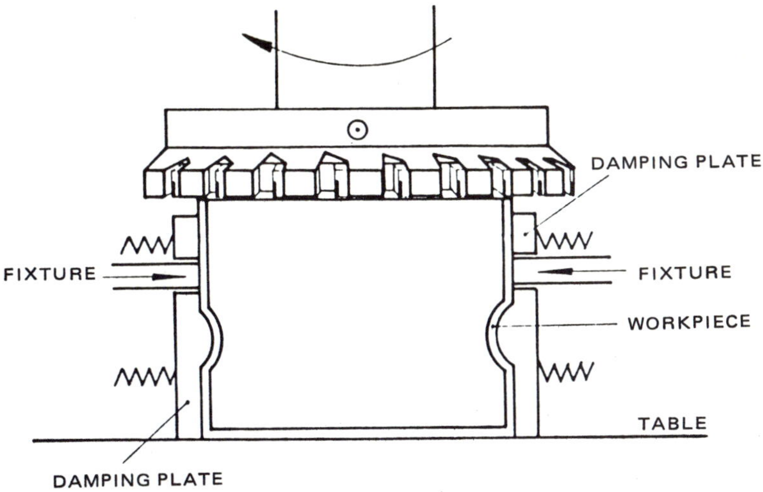

Fig. 9-12. The damping principle with damping plates[9]

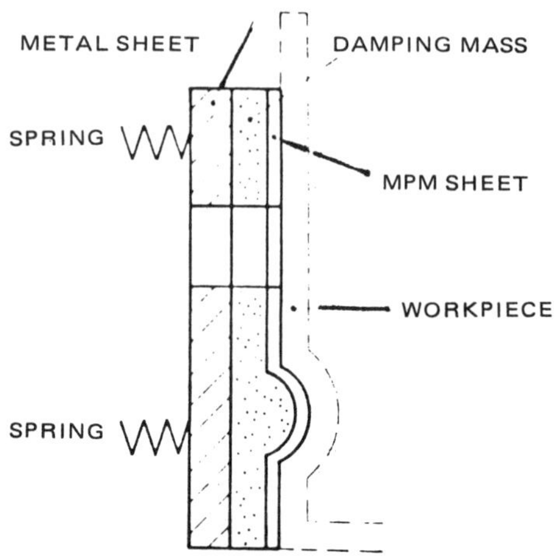

Fig. 9-13. The construction of a damping plate[9]

PNEUMATIC TOOLS

Most of the direct noise from the tool is due to pneumatic exhaust. The exhaust noise of almost all tools, except for newer models, exeeeds 90 dBA under both no-load and load conditions. The pneumatic tool industry was engaged in an increased power per pound race in the early sixties, which lead to an increase in tool noise. This complicates the situation greatly. There are, however, several methods for quieting exhaust noise.

1. Piped away exhaust
2. Expansion volume (muffler)
3. Diffusion at exit
4. Tortuous path

A pneumatic tool can and will make more noise when it is not in proper operating condition. One of the main causes of tool degeneration is water in the air lines. This can be corrected by air dryers and water traps. A regular maintenance program for pneumatic tools should be maintained. All rotary tools should also be checked for proper operating speeds. A tool which is being operated in a higher rpm range than that for which it was designed will create higher noise levels.

The impacts of pneumatic chipping hammers on metal parts create one of the highest noise levels found within modern industry. In some cases, this noise may be reduced by placing a casting in a sandbox for cleaning. The following sound levels were reported for chipping on a metal casting in a recent experiment by the U.S. Bureau of Mines:

Casting Placement	*dBA*
On concrete floor	113
On sand bed	105
One-half immersed in sand	101
Immersed to top in sand	98
Under sand	94

GEARS

Geared systems may be extremely noisy. Gears consist of assemblies of toothed wheels used for the purpose of torque conversion, speed change, or power distribution. The main sources of noise in geared systems are:

1. Impact caused by tooth contacts
2. Mechanical imbalance of the gear assembly
3. Friction due to the contact motion of the tooth
4. Variation of radial forces
5. Air and oil pocketing

Some of the principles used for reducing noise in gear systems are:

1. Selection of a suitable type of gear (for instance, a helical gear is quieter than a spur gear, and a worm gear is still quieter, but is restricted to low speeds).
2. Accuracy of manufacturing (high accuracy in all gear parameters results in quieter gear systems).
3. Detuning (when the operational frequency of the gear assembly coincides with the natural frequency of the structural members, resonance takes place, amplifying the noise; to avoid resonance, the structural members are detuned to other frequencies by either stiffening or mass loading).

4. Damping (introduced by using gear material of high internal damping).
5. Vibration isolation.
6. Enclosing the gear assembly (with particular attention given to cooling and heat transfer requirements).

CONCLUDING COMMENTS

The preceeding outline of noise control engineering provided basic information designed to acquaint the hearing conservationist with techniques which are employed to solve industrial noise problems. This background is important in order that hearing conservation and noise control programs of an industry may be properly coordinated. While these two elements of an industrial program both strive to achieve the common goal of protecting workers' hearing, the difference in talents required for their implementation should be recognized. Noise problems involving machine design should be handled by an engineer who possesses a background not only in industrial processes, but also has specialized training in noise control. An audiometric technician who attempts to design noise control measures without an engineering background may encounter technical problems which he is not capable of handling and also incur unnecessary personal liability. Even noise solutions which appear to be simple may reveal overlooked design requirements. For example, the installation of a small pneumatic muffler may cost only $10 and require five minutes to install. But the installation of even this simple measure without knowledge of machine backpressure requirements and air system contaminant contents can be dangerous! One case study indicates that one muffler installed on an unfiltered air line became clogged, blew off the machine and caused injury to an employee. There are numerous stories where the installation of mufflers with excessive back pressure rendered a machine inoperable.

For individuals who have the responsibility of developing noise control engineering solutions, specialized training is recommended. The following is a partial list of universities which offer several noise control courses in their curriculum:

Purdue University
Georgia Institute of Technology
Pennsylvania State University
North Carolina State University
Massachusetts Institute of Technology

Several short courses on noise control engineering are periodically offered throughout the United States. A few of the sponsors are:

Institute on Noise Control, Inc.
Bethlehem, PA 18017
Mr. J. H. Botsford (Dir.)

Purdue University
West Lafayette, IN 47901
Dr. M. J. Crocker (Mech. Eng.)

Bolt Beranck & Newman, Inc.
Cambridge, MA 02138
Mr. L. N. Miller (Principal Cons.)

Institute of Noise Control Engineering
Poughkeepsie, NY 12601
Dr. G. C. Maling (Secy.)

Georgia Institute of Technology
Atlanta, GA 30332
Dr. C. R. Bragdon (Arch.)

Bruel & Kjaer Instruments, Inc.
Cleveland, OH 44142
Mr. A. J. Schneider (B & K Inst.)

Massachusetts Institute of Technology
Cambridge, MA 02139
Dr. R. H. Lyon (Mech. Eng.)

Michigan Technical University
Houghton, MI 49931
Dr. H. W. Lord

North Carolina State University
Raleigh, NC 27607
Dr. F. D. Hart (Mech. Engr.)

Pennsylvania State University
University Park, PA 16802
Mr. J. H. Stevens (Cont. Ed.)

As basic introductory texts on noise control, the reader is referred to references 11 through 15. More specialized and advanced information may be found in references 16 through 22. Reference 23 covers the management aspects of an industrial noise control program. Also of interest is a series of reports published by the Southeast Acoustics Institute, Atlanta, GA, covering noise control solutions for the metal products, food, pulp and paper, textile, rubber and plastics, chemical and petroleum, and wood products industries.

REFERENCES

1. Harvey, S. G. and Oliver, C. C., "Classification and Performance of Commercial Vibration Isolators," Proceedings of *Inter-Noise 72,* 133-137, 1972.
2. Bell, L. H., *Fundamentals of Industrial Noise Control,* Harmony Publications, Trumbull, CT, 1973.
3. Sanders, G. J., "Silencers: Their Design and Application," *Sound and Vibration,* 2:2, 6-13, February 1968.
4. Jorgensen, Ed., *Fan Engineering,* 7th Edition, Buffalo Forge Company, Buffalo, NY, 1970.
5. Lord, H. W.; Evensen, H. A.; Canada, I. C.; and Palmer, M., "Effects of Modifications of Man Cooler Fans on Thermal and Noise Environments," Proceedings of NOISEXPO, 65-67, April 30–May 2, 1975.
6. Crede, C. E., "Principles of Vibration Control," Chapter 12, *Handbook of Noise Control,* edited by C. M. Harris, 12-26, McGraw-Hill, 1957.
7. Storment, J. W. and Pelton, H. K., "A Practical Approach to Noise Control in a Large Manufacturing Plant," Proceedings of NOISEXPO 1975, 207-218.
8. Handley, J. M., "Noise–The Third Pollution," IAC Bulletin 6.0011.0, 1973.
9. Karlsson, S. O., "Noise Reduction When Milling Thin Walled Workpieces," Proceedings of *Inter-Noise 76,* 37-42, April 5-7, 1976.
10. L. S. Goodfriend Associates, "Noise from Industrial Plants," U.S. EPA No. NT10300.2; December 31, 1971.
11. Thumann, A. and Miller, R. K., *Secrets of Noise Control,* Third Edition, Fairmont Press, Atlanta, GA, 1979.

12. Yerges, L. F., *Sound, Noise and Vibration Control,* Van Nostrand Reinhold, New York, 1969.
13. Peterson, A. P. G. and Gross, E. E., Jr., "Handbook of Noise Measurement," General Radio Company, 1972.
14. Rettinger, M., *Acoustics, Room Design and Noise Control,* Chemical Publishing Co., New York, 1968.
15. Egan, *Concepts in Architectural Acoustics,* McGraw-Hill, New York.
16. Harris, C. M., *Handbook on Noise Control,* McGraw-Hill, New York, 1957.
17. Kinsler, L. E. and Frey, A. R., *Fundamentals of Acoustics,* Second Edition, Wiley, 1962.
18. Beranek, L. L., *Noise Reduction,* McGraw-Hill, New York, 1960.
19. Beranek, L. L., *Noise and Vibration Control,* McGraw-Hill, New York, 1971.
20. Kryter, K. D., *Effects of Noise on Man,* Academic Press, New York, 1970.
21. Morse, P.M. and Ingard, K.U., *Theoretical Acoustics,* McGraw-Hill, 1968.
22. Skudrzyk, E., *Simple and Complex Vibratory Systems,* Pennsylvania State University Press, 1968.
23. Miller, R. K., *Handbook of Industrial Noise Management,* Fairmont Press, 1976.

Glossary

1. **Acuity** – In this sense pertains to the sensitivity of hearing.
2. **Air Conduction** – The process by which sound is conducted to the inner ear (cochlea) via the air medium.
3. **Ambient Noise Level** – The audible alterations in air pressure caused by the everpresent noise of the environment. It is usually a composite of sounds from varying sources at varying distances.
4. **ANSI (1969)** – American National Standards Institute.
5. **ASA (1951)** – American Standards Association.
6. **Attenuate** – To reduce in amount as in audiometry by turning the hearing level dial in units of 10 or five decibels in order to obtain a threshold of hearing.
7. **Audible Range** – The frequency range over which normal ears hear approximately 20 cycles through 20,000 cycles. Above the range of 20,000 cycles, the term ultrasonic is used. Below 20 cycles, the term infra- or subsonic is used.
8. **Audiogram** – A record of hearing loss or hearing level measured at several different frequencies–usually 500 to 6,000 cycles. The audiogram may be presented graphically or numerically.
9. **Audiologist** – A person trained in the specialized problems of hearing and deafness. A hearing scientist.
10. **Audiometer** – A signal generator or instrument for measuring objectively the sensitivity of hearing in decibels or intensity, frequency or pitch.
11. **Audiometric Curves** – (1) Ascending: greater loss in low frequencies. (2) Descending: greater loss in high frequencies. (3) Abrupt drop: change of 40 dB or more in one octave. (4) Basin: greater loss in middle frequencies. (5) Dip:

a depression of 10 dB or more and subsequent return to former level. (6) Peak: elevation of 10 dB or more and subsequent return to former level. (7) Unilateral: a greater amount of loss in one ear than in the other, usually of 10 dB or more at three or more frequencies. (8) Bilateral-Symmetrical: similar threshold levels at all frequencies.

12. **Audiometric Technician** – A person who is trained and qualified to administer audiometric examinations.
13. **Automatic Audiometry** – The method most often used for testing large numbers of persons. It eliminates the need for a technician, ostensibly, except to begin the test. The subject controls the presentation of sound and records his response.
14. **Aural** – Of or pertaining to the ear or hearing.
15. **A-Weighted Sound Level (dBA)** – A number in decibels, which is read from a sound-level meter, when the meter is switched to its weighting labeled "A". The number approximately measures the relative noisiness or annoyance level of many common sounds. (The human ear is less efficient at low and high sound frequencies than at medium or speech-range frequencies. In order to obtain a single number for the level of a noise containing a wide range of frequencies, in a manner which represents the ear's response, it is necessary to reduce or weight the effects of the low and high frequencies with respect to the medium frequencies. The resultant sound level is said to be A-weighted.)
16. **Binaural Hearing** – Refers to hearing with both ears.
17. **Calibrate** – To check an audiometer for uniformity or accuracy. It may be done biologically and electronically.
18. **Cerumen** – Ear wax.
19. **Cochlea** – The auditory part of the internal ear, shaped like a snail shell. It contains the basilar membrane on which the end organs of the auditory nerve are distributed.
20. **Conduction Deafness** – An impairment of hearing due to the failure of vibrations to be transmitted to the cochlea. This type of deafness can often be corrected medically or surgically.

21. **Damage-Risk Criterion** – A statement of noise levels (including frequency, duration, intermittency, and other factors) which if exceeded are likely to cause permanent hearing loss to a specified minimum degree.
22. **Deaf** – The term used to describe a person who has lost his hearing before the speech patterns were established.
23. **Deafened** – A person who has lost his ability to hear after normal speech patterns were established.
24. **Decibel (dB)** – One-tenth of a bel. Sound intensity is measured in decibels. The zero on the decibel scale is based on the lowest sound level that the healthy, unimpaired human ear can detect (re: 0.0002 dyne/cm^2). Decibels are not linear units, but representative points on a sharply rising (exponential) curve. Thus, 100 decibels represent 10 billion times as much acoustic energy as one decibel.
25. **DOT** – Department of Transportation.
26. **Ear Defenders** – Or simply plugs or muffs designed to keep noxious noise from the ear to preserve hearing.
27. **EPA** – Environmental Protection Agency.
28. **Frequency** – The number of vibrations expressed in cycles per second or Hertz. It is sometimes called pitch or the highness or lowness of sound. High frequencies damage more easily than low frequencies in noise-induced hearing loss.
29. **Hearing Conservation** – The prevention or minimizing of noise-induced deafness through the use of hearing protection devices and the control of noise through engineering methods.
30. **Hearing Level** – Formerly called "hearing loss," the deviation in decibels of an individual's threshold from the zero reference of the audiometer.
31. **HEW** – Health, Education and Welfare Department.
32. **High Frequency Loss** – Refers to a deficit starting with 2,000 Hz and beyond.
33. **Interrupter Switch** – Usually called the "presenter switch" because it permits the stimulus to be presented or cut off from the earphones, but it leaves the audiometer circuits

in operation making it possible to change the frequency and intensity level of the tone.

34. **ISO (1964)** – International Standards Organization.
35. **Loudness** – The intensive attribute of an auditory sensation, in psychological terms of which sounds may be ordered on a scale extending from soft to loud. Loudness depends primarily upon the sound pressure of the stimulus, but it also depends upon the frequency and wave form of the stimulus.
36. **Malingerer** – One who pretends deafness or other abnormalities.
37. **Masking** – The stimulation of one ear of a subject by controlled noise to prevent his hearing with that ear the tone or signal given to the other ear. This procedure is used where there is at least 15 to 20 dB difference in the two ears.
38. **Microbar, Dyne Per Square Centimeter** – A unit of pressure commonly used in acoustics. One microbar is equal to one dyne per square centimeter. Note: The term "bar" properly denotes a pressure of 10^6 dynes per square centimeter.
39. **Monaural Hearing** – Refers to hearing with one ear only.
40. **Noise** – Any unwanted sound.
41. **Noise-Induced Hearing Loss** – The terminology used to refer to the slowly progressive inner ear hearing loss that results from exposure to continuous noise over a long period of time as contrasted to acoustic trauma or physical injury to the ear.
42. **Noise Reduction Coefficient (NRC)** – A measure of the acoustical absorption performance of a material, calculated by averaging its sound absorption coefficients at 250, 500, 1000, and 2000 Hz, expressed to the nearest integral multiple of 0.05.
43. **NIOSH** – National Institute of Occupational Safety and Health.
44. **Nonauditory Effects of Noise** – Refers to stress, fatigue, work efficiency, and performance effects of loud noise that is continuous.

45. **Octave** – The interval between two sounds having a basic frequency ratio of two. For example, there are eight octaves on the keyboard of a standard piano.
46. **Octave Band** – All of the components, in a sound spectrum, the frequencies of which are between two sine wave components separated by an octave.
47. **Octave Band Sound Pressure Level** – The integrated sound pressure level of only those sine-wave components in a specified octave band, for a noise or sound having a wide spectrum.
48. **Organ of Corti** – A structure resting on the basilar membrane within the cochlear duct (scala media). It contains the essential sensory elements of hearing, the hair cells, together with their supporting cells. The function of the hair cells is to convert sound pressure waves into nerve impulses which are transmitted by way of the VIII cranial nerve to the brain. It is the end organ of hearing.
49. **OSHA** – Occupational Safety Health Agency.
50. **Ossicle** – A small bone, any member of a chain of three bones from the outer membrane of the tympanum (eardrum) to the membrane covering the oval window of the inner ear: Malleus, Incus, Stapes.
51. **Otologist** – A physician who has specialized in surgery and diseases of the ear.
52. **Otosclerosis** – Hardening of the ear caused by a growth of bony tissue about the foot plate of the stapes and the oval window of the inner ear. It results in a gradual loss of hearing. Surgery can often correct this.
53. **Pitch** – A listener's perception of the frequency of a pure tone. The higher the frequency, the higher the pitch.
54. **Presbycusis** – The hearing loss due to age and the loss of nerve capacity. It is believed by some to be the degeneration of the nerve cells due to ordinary wear and tear on their structure as a result of environmental noise.
55. **Psychogenic Deafness** – Deafness originating in or produced by the mental reaction of an individual to his physical or social environment. It is sometimes called functional deafness or feigned deafness.

56. **Reliability** – The repeatability of threshold responses within ± 5dB.
57. **Sensorineural Deafness** – Nerve deafness or the lack of sensitivity of the auditory mechanism in the cochlea. This was formerly called inner ear impairment or perceptive deafness.
58. **Semicircular Canals** – The special organs of balance that are closely associated with the hearing mechanism and the VIII cranial nerve. Vestibular Mechanism.
59. **Sine Wave** – A sound wave, audible as a pure tone, in which the sound pressure is a sinusoidal function of time.
60. **Sociocusis** – Refers to both the progressive loss of hearing due to the aging process (presbycusis) and the loss due to disease or noise exposure in modern society.
61. **Sound** – The sensation produced through the organs of hearing–usually by vibrations transmitted in a material medium, commonly air.
62. **Sound Level Meter and Octave Band Analyzer** – Instruments for measuring sound pressure levels in decibels referenced to 0.0002 microbars. Readings can also be made in specific octave bands, usually beginning at 75 Hz and continuing through 10,000 Hz.
63. **Sound Pressure Level** – In decibels, 20 times the logarithm to the base 10 of the ratio of the pressure of this sound to the reference pressure. The reference pressure shall be explicitly stated (2×10^{-4} microbar or 0.0002 dyne/cm^2).
64. **Speech Discrimination Test** – A measurement of hearing acuity by the administration of a carefully controlled list of words. The identification of correct responses is evaluated in terms of norms established by the average performance of normal listeners.
65. **Temporary Threshold Shift (TTS)** – The hearing loss suffered as the result of noise exposure, all or part of which is recovered during an arbitrary period of time when one is removed from the noise. It accounts for the necessity of checking hearing acuity at least 16 hours after a noise exposure.

66. **Threshold** – The point at which a person just begins to notice the tone is becoming audible.
67. **Tinnitus** – A ringing, buzzing or roaring sound in the ears.
68. **Tone Deafness** – The inability to make a close discrimination between fundamental tones close together in pitch.
69. **Tort** – A wrongful act for which civil damage suits can be brought.
70. **Ultra and Infra Sonics** – Above (ultra) or below (infra) the frequency range of human auditory acuity.
71. **Validity** – True baseline thresholds having legal efficacy or force.
72. **Walsh-Healey Act** – Formerly known as Government Contracts Act. Applied to industry when executing Government work.
73. **Williams-Javitts Act** – An act to standardize Worker's Compensation laws.

Appendix A

Model Industrial Audiometric Technician Course (2-½ Days)

I. **Introduction to Course**
   A. Course content.
   B. Noise as an environmental pollutant.
   C. Social aspects of noise and its effects.
   D. Importance of hearing conservation in industry.

II. **Responsibilities and Limitations of the Audiometric Technician**
   A. Obtaining accurate, reliable hearing thresholds.
   B. Record keeping (Storage, etc.).
   C. Distribution and proper fitting of ear protection devices following measurement of ear canal size.
   D. Insuring proper calibration of all instrumentation and test chamber.
   E. Keeping abreast with changes and techniques in governmental regulations (refresher course every year or two).
   F. Referral to professional diagnosticians.
   G. Insure review of audiograms is completed and that recommendations are followed.

H. Be able to take cursory and/or basic SPL measures.
   1. Being aware of the nature of Pure-tone air conduction testing.
   2. Limited training: no diagnosis nor test information to employee.
   3. Medico-legal aspects in workmen's compensation.

III. **Film: "Death Be Not Loud."** Discussion of film following presentation.

IV. **Physical Basis of Hearing**
   A. Slide presentation of gross anatomy and physiology showing the sound pathways.
   B. Explanation of energy change from airborne acoustical to mechanical to hydraulic to electrochemical (neurological).
   C. Physiology of outer, middle and inner ear mechanisms.
      1. Detailed description of cochlear function.
      2. Description of central auditory pathways.
      3. Vestibular involvement.
   D. Etiology of hearing impairment.
      1. Conductive loss (external and middle ear: cerumen, cholesteatoma, otitis media, otosclerosis, etc.).
      2. Sensorineural loss (noise induced, traumatic vs. noise induced, Meniere's, labyrinthitis, tinnitus, vertigo, presbycusis, T.T.S., etc.).
      3. Mixed loss (ossicular chain disruption and sensorineural loss—explosion or blow to head), sociocusis, etc.

V. **Non-End-Organ Effects of Noise**
   A. Acuity vs. perception (comprehending hearing).
   B. Protective and interpretive functions of hearing and stress factors.
   C. Basics of Central Nervous System areas stimulated and how they affect the entire body.
   D. Auditory overload and disruption of higher cortical functions.
   E. Psychological effects: work situation, social and personal life.

VI. **Instrumentation (Physics of Sound and Its Measurement) Definitions for Discussion:**

A. Sound
B. Noise
C. SPL
D. Intensity, loudness (see F.)
E. Frequency (Hz), pitch
F. Decibel (dBA)
G. Threshold (HL vs. SL)
H. Octave band
I. Acuity
J. Attenuate
K. Octave band analyzer
L. Impact noise (impulsive)
M. Damage risk criteria
N. Temporary threshold shift (T.T.S.)
O. Audiometric zero
P. Infra sound
Q. Ultrasonics
R. Steady-state noise
S. Ambient noise (background noise)
T. ISO – 1964, ANSI – 1969
U. Audiometer
V. L10, 50, 90 levels

VII. **Demonstration of Instrumentation**

A. Sound level meter and octave band analyzer
B. Dosimeter
C. Calibrator for instrumentation

VIII. **Acoustical Engineering and Noise Control**

A. OSHA Requirements
   1. 90 dBA/8 hours
   2. Exposure time
   3. Necessity for engineering
   4. Administrative controls
B. Noise Generation
   1. Vibration
   2. Air Noise

C. Approaches to Noise Control
   1. Source
   2. Path
   3. Receiver
D. Engineering Solutions
   1. Sound Barriers
      a. Enclosures
      b. Walls
      c. Curtains
   2. Sound Absorbers
      a. Room Acoustics
      b. Inside Enclosures
      c. Bafflers, Ceilings
   3. Vibration Damping
      a. Surface Damping
      b. Increase Mass
      c. Increase Stiffness
   4. Vibration Isolation
      a. Spring Mounts
      b. Rubber Resilient Mounts
      c. Flexible Couplings
      d. Rubber Bumpers or Cushions
   5. Mufflers
      a. Pneumatic
      b. Fan Inlet/Outlet
      c. Engine Exhaust
   6. Substitution
      a. Larger, slower machines for smaller, faster ones.
      b. Step dies for single operation dies.
      c. Presses for Hammers.
      d. Rotating shears for square shears.
      e. Hydraulic for mechanical presses.
      f. Belt drives for gears.
      g. Compression for impact riveting.
      h. Welding for riveting.
      i. Hot for cold working.
      j. Pressing for rolling or forging.

7. Maintenance
   a. Replacement or adjustment of worn and loose or unbalanced parts of machines.
   b. Lubrication of machine parts and use of cutting oils.
   c. Properly shaped and sharpened cutting tools.

IX. Audiometer Function, Care and Calibration

A. Description of audiometers (in general) and manual, limited frequency audiometers vs. self-recording (automatic audiometer).
   1. On-off switch.
   2. Frequency dial (indicator).
   3. Interrupter switch (tone interrupter–normally on-normally off).
   4. Plug and cord vs. battery operation.
   5. TDH-39 vs. otocup (Auraldomes).
   6. Ear selection (red, right, round, etc.).
   7. Biological and electronic calibration.

B. Techniques
   1. Preparing subjects (after otoscopic inspection).
   2. Test instructions.
   3. Seating subject.
   4. Placing earphones (head set).
   5. Testing techniques.
      a. 1K, 2K, 3K, 4K, and 6K then 500 Hz. Right ear first, then left at same frequencies. Retest 1000 Hz in right ear for test–retest reliability ±5 dB.
      b. Response criteria (50% to determine threshold).
      c. Recording responses (graph vs. bar graph), numerical or graphical.
      d. Limits of audiometer (intensity and frequency).

X. Practicum (Supervised)

A. Testing each other.

B. Testing on master audiometer.

XI. Review of Audiograms and Additional Practice
Types of Audiograms, Their Significance and Interpretation and/or When to Refer

XII. Problems of Hearing Testing (Pitfalls)

A. Subject variables (language barrier, understanding instructions, etc.).
B. Tester variables (technique, rhythm, eye contact, etc.).
C. Instrumentation variables (improper calibration, standing waves, collapsed canal).
(Test questions: audiometer, techniques and problems)

XIII. Hearing Protection

A. Plugs
B. Muffs
C. Valves
D. Wool
E. Cotton
F. Molds
G. Measurement technique for fitting proper protective devices.
H. Attenuation properties of each device.
I. Hygiene (ear protection, care and aural cleanliness).
J. Contraindications to fitting: allergies, external otitis, impacted cerumen, middle ear infections, perforations, etc.

XIV. Medical-Legal Aspects

A. Historical Perspective
Walsh-Healey Act
Williams-Steiger Act
OSHA
NIOSH
EPA
ANSI (delineation of functions)
B. Workmen's Compensation
Basic History
Statutory allowances
Tort claims

C. Williams-Javits Act
Results obtained
Results expected
Effect on Occupational Hearing Loss

D. Legal responsibilities of Audiometric Technicians. Court appearance. Method used to obtain electrical calibration reading certification; biological calibration by log entries.

XV. Otoscopic Inspection

A. Slides from Shambaugh's Surgery of the Ear, 1967 (Normal vs. Pathological)
Slides illustrating pneumo-message (Otologist)

B. Techniques of inspection

C. Hygiene (otoscopic speculae)

D. When to refer (presence of any ear abnormality)

E. Types of Otoscopes

XVI. Record Keeping

A. In-plant vs. computer storage (tape and microfilm)

B. Case history (detailed discussion of relevancy of past and present history)

C. Corrections on audiogram and/or history (in ink, signed, tester number)

D. Relevance of 14-hour non-noise exposure (less than 80 dBA) loss of validity of baseline and/or follow-up audiograms

E. Difference between baseline and follow-up audiograms

F. Importance of updating Hx on follow-up audiogram

G. Letter to previous employer

XVII. Role of the Industrial Nurse in Hearing Conservation

A. Interprofessional communication role: Doctor, Industrial Hygienist, Audiologist, etc.

B. Practical suggestions relative to data taking, employee education re hearing protection and testing

XVIII. Review of Both Days and Final Written Examination

XIX. Review of Examination Papers

XX. Additional Practicum As Needed

Published: September 30, 1974

Prepared for joint course presentation: Florida Technological University, Orlando, Florida, and Hearex Corporation, Tampa, Florida, by:

David F. Barr, Ph.D.
Thomas A. Mullin, Ph.D.
Richard K. Miller, B.S.
and Cecil E. Kline

NOTES

NOTES

NOTES

NOTES

NOTES

NOTES

NOTES

NOTES

NOTES

NOTES